WALK!

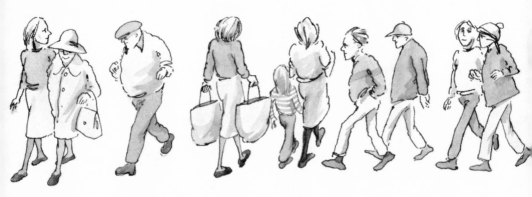

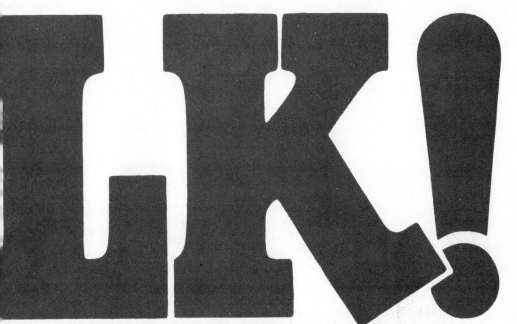

LK!

IT COULD CHANGE YOUR LIFE...

A HANDBOOK
BY JOHN MAN

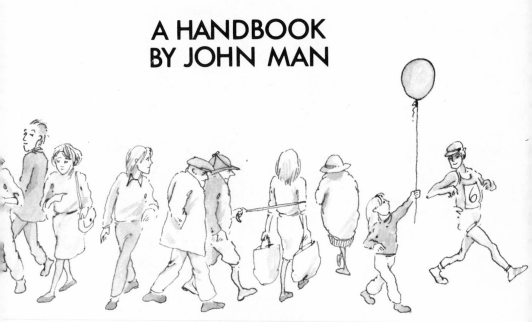

PADDINGTON PRESS LTD

NEW YORK & LONDON

Library of Congress Cataloging in Publication Data
Man, John.
    Walk! It could change your life.

    Bibliography: p.
    Includes index.
    1.   Physical fitness.   2. Walking.   I.   Title.
GV481.M34   796.5'1   78-23655
ISBN 0 448 22685 5 (U.S. and Canada only)
ISBN 0 7092 0515 5

Filmset in England by SX Composing Ltd., Rayleigh, Essex.
Printed and bound in the United States.
Designed by Colin Lewis
Wash drawings by Julia Whatley
Photo research by Susan de la Plain and Karen Moline

In the United States
PADDINGTON PRESS
Distributed by
GROSSET & DUNLAP

In the United Kingdom
PADDINGTON PRESS

In Canada
Distributed by
RANDOM HOUSE OF CANADA LTD.

In Southern Africa
Distributed by
ERNEST STANTON (PUBLISHERS) (PTY.) LTD.

In Australia and New Zealand
Distributed by
A. H. & A. W. REED

Contents

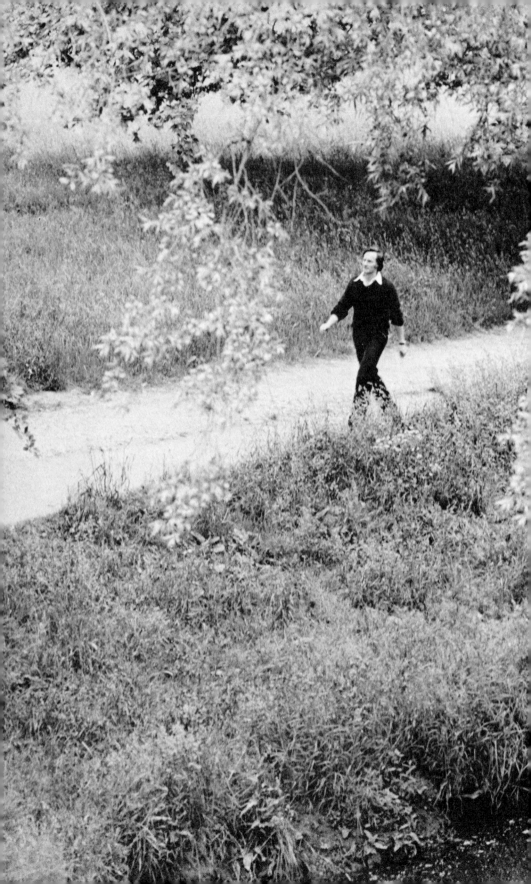

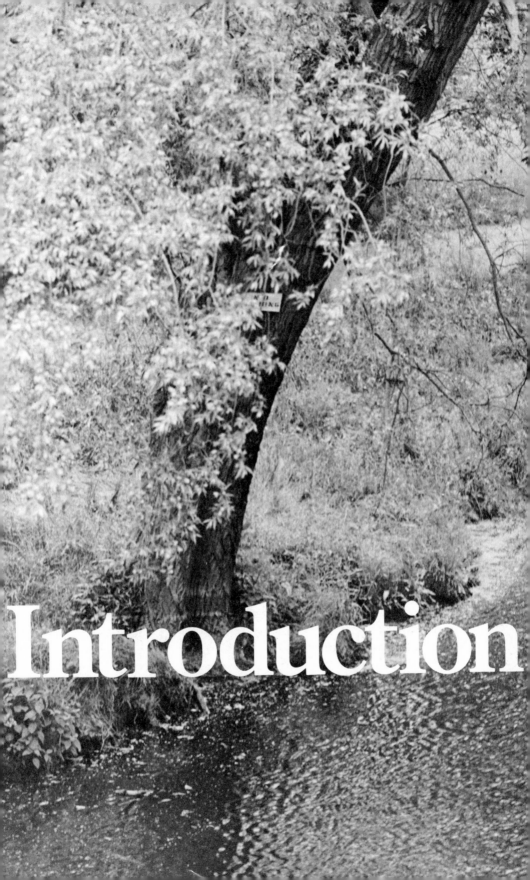

Introduction

Introduction

*"Something hidden. Go and find it. Go and look
 behind the ranges —
Something lost behind the ranges. Lost and
 waiting for you. Go!"*

Rudyard Kipling

THE MESSAGE OF THIS book is a simple one: for basic fitness
and emotional release, get walking. Though the rhythm of
our age is beaten out by running feet and it may seem bold to
say so, you do not *have* to run.

There are many memories I could use to dramatize the contrast between running and walking. Here are just two:

I am in the Oxford University Parks, near my home, a mile
from the center of the city. The Parks, ninety acres gently
edged by the River Cherwell, form a landscape of rare beauty,
containing some five hundred different species of trees in
groves scattered across and around the fields and sports areas.
It is a perfect summer's day. I am running, surrounded by
sights and sounds of familiar charm. To my right, a cricket
match is in stately progress. Ahead of me, on the river, adept
students and incompetent tourists pole punts. Arpeggios of
laughter ripple up from the river banks. Children play on
newly felled elms, diseased giants now being replaced. I know
all this is there, but I sense none of it. My rasping breath
drowns the laughter, sweat stings my eyes, my heart hammers
at my rib cage. I am locked in a world of my own sensations,
and outside me another world slips by into oblivion . . .

It is a fall day in the western Catskills. Angy, my wife, and
I are staying with a journalist friend, Keith Johnson, deep in
the rolling woodlands a few miles from the Delaware River that
divides New York State from Pennsylvania. The surrounding
forests are still glowing with the last dazzling displays of reds,
yellows, browns and purples that make upstate New York
autumns so startling to newcomers like ourselves. We walk,
the three of us, down through steeply sloping woodlands toward a forest track that will take us several miles deeper into
the mountains. An inches-thick carpet of leaves and twigs

8

crackle and rustle underfoot. Unaccountably I ask Keith to explain the US Constitution. As we hit the track and begin to head out past the few clapboard farm buildings, he begins to humor me. The conversation lasts, oh, two or three hours, with frequent diversions to consider other vital matters – like the difficulties of making maple syrup the traditional way (you have to boil fifty gallons of sap to make one gallon of syrup), and the way the forest has recolonized the stone-walled mowings of the early settlers. At one high point we look back over range upon range of flowing forests, fall colors merging into a misty distance. Years later I remember almost nothing of the US Constitution and not all I should about local lore; but the feel of that day is woven into our three lives. We shall always be linked by the special sort of shared delight that can be acquired only on foot.

No need, though, for mere effusiveness. I have reason as well as emotion on my side.

I am getting on toward 40 now. I have always liked to think I keep fairly fit. At university, when I used to throw the javelin in a desultory way, I got into the habit of working out with weights, and I have done it on and off ever since. I can play a hard, if wild, game of tennis.

But still, in recent years, the facts about health across the western world bothered me, in particular the statistics on heart attacks. In 1977 in the US there were one and half million "coronary events," as the medical profession euphemistically terms crises of the heart and circulatory systems. Half a million people died from heart attacks. Among American males between 33 and 65 coronary heart disease causes one-third of all deaths. In the United Kingdom the figures are less dramatic among the population at large: 50,000 die of heart attacks each year. But one in three members of the Institute of Directors dies of a heart attack before reaching retirement.

Sure, there are studies enough to show that we do not have to suffer this way. Coronary heart disease is a relatively "new" disease, the product of our peculiar life style. Among the Masai of East Africa, for whom daily exercise is a regular part of a cattle-herding existence, heart disease is virtually unknown. And in the US, the running revolution has been followed by (and most doctors would say has "led to") a small but signifi-

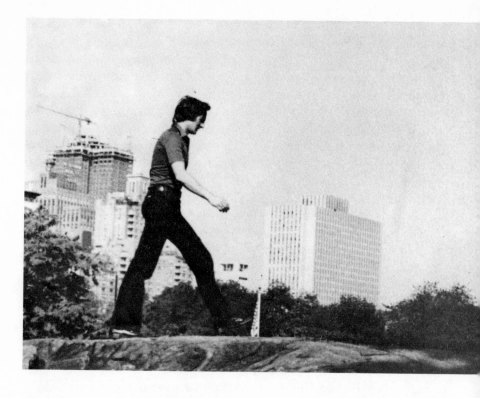

cant decrease in the incidence of heart attacks. There is no
known case of a practicing marathoner succumbing to a heart
attack, and it has even been claimed that you can make yourself virtually immune from heart disease by running thirty
miles or more a week.

OK. I believe it. I am appalled by the figures. I believe something can be done. I believe I should plan for my own health in
middle age. But nevertheless somewhere along the line I have
switched off. I don't *want* to run thirty miles a week. It is very
tiring, it takes a large slice out of each day, and it's unsociable.
I don't want to spend so much of my life working to keep myself
alive that I am left with no time to live.

Of course, there are countless people who want to run, to be
super-fit, for any number of reasons – to feel a sense of achievement, to satisfy a strong competitive instinct, to live longer, to
live better, to express a talent. But not me. And not millions of
others who are put off by the strain of running and by the
holier-than-thou elitism of runners. There must, I thought, be
an easier way . . .

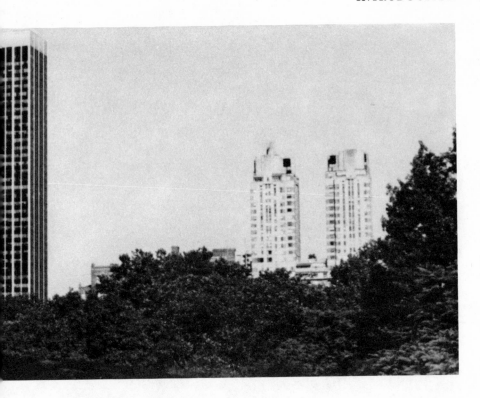

There is. Walking. If you are very unfit, even a stroll can count as exercise. I once met a New York cab driver who weighed 260 pounds. He had just started a walking program. It tired him to walk more than a hundred yards. For him, every pace demanded the expenditure of a significant amount of energy, but he knew that if he kept at it he could build up slowly and it would be worth the effort. But looking beyond that: if you walk regularly, if you walk for distance, if you walk fast, if you walk uphill, you can build exactly the same level of fitness as you can with a basic running program.

The advantages are many. You need no special equipment (unless you are backpacking), you won't suffer any undue injuries, you don't have to compete, no one will look at you if you're slow or overweight, and a variety of joys are yours for the choosing. Woods, hills, seashores, cities, friends, colleagues, the family – all offer delights that are largely excluded if you are simply a runner.

Keep pace with me and I'll show you.

Stepping Out

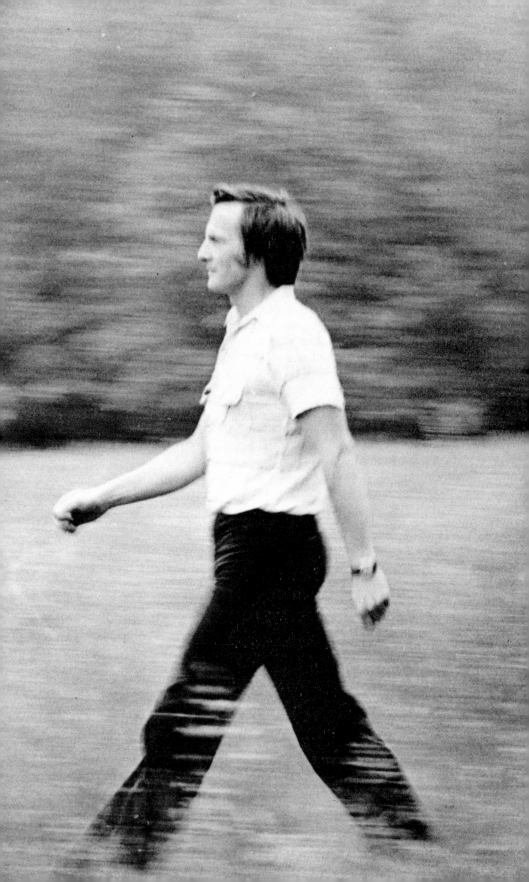

Stepping Out

AS A TEENAGER I used to read science fiction. A popular scenario of the times was of a future world in which mankind had evolved to such a state of technological achievement that legs had become unnecessary. People preferred to get around on antigravity devices and legs had atrophied away to minute residual appendages.

The idea provoked a certain fascination in the 1950s when postwar affluence promised a car in every garage. But it's a ridiculous notion. Walking still cements the fabric of our lives. Even the most sedentary of office workers must walk from house to car, from car to office and back again, and to accomplish this, he or she brings a full complement of bones and muscles into play.

There is certainly no evidence that the joys of mechanical transportation will ever overtake the joys of walking. In a 1973 survey by the President's Council on Physical Fitness and Sports, forty-four million adult Americans claimed they walked for exercise; over half of them said they went out daily or almost every day for at least twenty minutes per outing. Of those who claimed to do other exercises – bicycling, swimming, gymnastics, running – most said they went out less than once a week for less than twenty minutes. All in all, therefore, there are some three to four times as many regular walkers as runners in the US (depending on the figures you care to accept). Moreover, they exercise for precisely the same reasons as runners do: "It's good for my heart." "It keeps me slim." "It's good for me." One might justly conclude that America is not a nation of runners at all, but a nation of walkers.

Well, hardly a nation: only 55 percent of the population claim they take any exercise at all. Besides, the walkers don't publicize their activities very much and probably most of them are

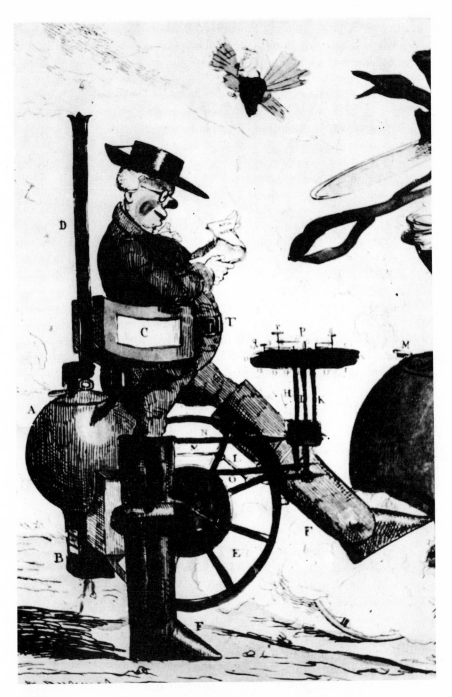

*"The Steam Walker": The English nineteenth-century cartoonist
George Cruikshank satirizes the idea of replacing legs with machinery.*

unaware of the good they're doing themselves, or of how much more good they *could* be doing themselves if they cared to increase their activity a little more. Hence the need for this book.

Starting from Scratch

Hence, too, the need to start from first principles. Walking is as easy as breathing, and just as vital; in fact, it's such a natural activity that it seems to go against the grain to analyze it. Yet it is both possible and necessary to do so. The variety of walks, for instance, is a minor study in itself. Desmond Morris in his book *Manwatching* light-heartedly identifies four types of walking styles:

1. The walk: the human being's normal basic gait of between three and four miles an hour. The healthy nonathlete can usually keep this up for several miles without too much trouble and the trained walker can cover enormous distances. (The greatest distance ever walked nonstop is 234 miles by Britain's Thomas Benson. He covered this distance around the Aintree Race Course in 1978. It took him four days and four nights.)

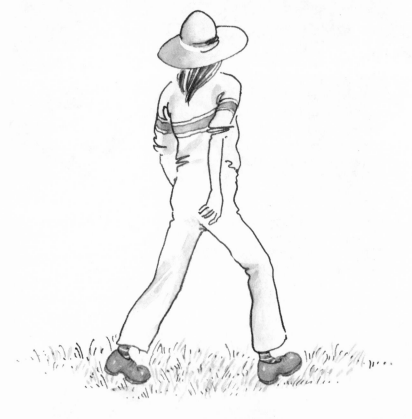

2. The hurry: a fast walk, adopted by anyone who is late for an appointment or rushing to catch a train after office hours. The arms bend, the shoulders move up and down, the hips wiggle, the pace stretches out. It's this action, much refined, that race walkers adopt. Some walkers can achieve speeds of over 9 MPH – faster than a comfortable running speed, but also far more demanding.

3. The stroll: the type of locomotion adopted by tourists, lovers, promenaders and thinkers. (The Peripatetics, the school of ancient Greek philosophers founded by Aristotle, took their name from the Greek word meaning "covered walk": they taught and discussed while strolling.)

4. The shuffle: the hobbling gait of the aged and the infirm, in which the feet are slid cautiously along the ground. Progression may be at a snail's pace, but at least the shuffler does eventually get where he wants to go and can keep active. As a child I remember an aged man, bent almost double with the burden of the years, who used to shuffle along the Kentish lanes, near my home. I never knew where he lived, but he was out every day. He looked well into his 90s. I remember my father saying: "He's been out every day as long as I can remember. I suppose he'll keep at it until he dies."

Walking thus represents a whole spectrum of movement and activity reflecting our abilities, age and health. Much of this book is an attempt to make you conscious of an activity that you so often unconsciously perform and to show what physical benefits can be made to flow from it; but before getting into the basics, I want to talk first about the other side to walking – the emotional one.

Something Good for Heart and Mind

People who walk for exercise usually enjoy walking for other reasons as well – they feel, in a vague sort of way, that it is good for them to do so, not only in a physical sense but in a spiritual one. It is hard to articulate clearly, but walking does something for both heart and mind. This finds expression in many different ways – in the family walk at the weekend, in the

"*I never met a human being whose humor was not the better for a walk.*"

Donald Culross Peattie, *The Joy of Walking*

early evening promenade common in Mediterranean countries, in walking with one's dog, in the lovers' stroll, in the determined step of the nature rambler. If you ask people why they walk and what they get out of it, their responses are usually naive in the extreme: "It's nice to get out and about." "A bit of fresh air does you good." But such phrases tell you virtually nothing about the real emotional reasons for going for a walk.

The prime impulse, it would seem, comes from the human need to move and to seek new, but not totally unfamiliar stimuli. Human beings are naturally restless creatures. We cannot keep still for very long. An average night's sleep involves some sixty to seventy movements – not because the body seeks more comfortable places in bed, but because the limbs themselves become uncomfortable if they remain motionless for more than a few minutes. Human beings have an average concentration span of about ninety minutes. But the attention span of any muscle is much less than this, as any concert hall or conference room testifies. Beneath the rapt attention is a mass of tiny motions. People scratch their noses and joggle their knees; they shift their weight from one buttock to another; they cross and uncross their legs. One habit of mine is to scrape my heel on the ground. I sometimes catch myself doing this during a long lunch or a conference, and am always amazed to realize that I must have been doing it for many minutes, completely unconsciously. Guardsmen who have to remain standing for long periods of time learn to wriggle their toes or tense and untense their muscles, to ensure that there is enough movement to keep the circulation going without breaking the apparent rigidity of their pose. None of these involuntary or voluntary movements necessarily indicate boredom; they simply reflect the fact that there is a very strict limit to how much inactivity our muscles can take. We are literally driven to action.

Impelled to motion, there are countless ways in which we express ourselves physically. What is so special about walking?

It is easy, controlled and rhythmical. It uses muscles for precisely the task they have evolved to do. Energy output can be exactly controlled and the ground is covered at a swinging pace that is fast enough to be rewarding, yet slow enough to be undemanding.

But there are deeper answers than this – some of them external, involving a special relationship between the walker and the outside world; and still others that are deeply internal ones. Just what is it that makes walking so good for heart and mind?

When I was last in Washington, I made a point of talking to Stewart Udall, former secretary of the interior under President Kennedy in the early 1960s. At that time he had a driving professional and personal interest, as Kennedy had, in promoting a sense of national vigor. In Udall's case this was combined with a passion for the American wilderness – in particular the national parks, for which he was responsible. He has walked mountains, forests and plains, both alone and with family or friends. It is a passion he still retains, at 58, as a senior partner in a Washington law firm.

"When I start walking, I find myself actually relaxing," he said. "The strain drops away from me. I think walking is a way of closing the mind off from one's problems. Your senses become tuned to the natural world. The pace of that world and of your own motion is very different and very soothing compared to the world you've just left. The mental relaxation involved is tremendous. You can get it in the same way with gathering wood, gardening and other things, but getting back to nature is one of the great tonics. A city is meant to be civilized, and yet with the pollution and the noise, I find it very *un*civilized. I have a rather low tolerance and I instinctively try to turn it off. I can do that when I'm out walking."

I had a similar conversation with George Zoebelein, chairman of the Appalachian Trail Conference and a senior partner of an accounting firm. "I find that being able to get away from the pressures of the city provides me with a feeling of emotional well-being," he told me. "The burdens of the week slip away from me as I take to the trails. It's a relaxation response. It's not particularly conscious. In the springtime I look at the flowers, not necessarily being able to identify each species but simply enjoying the beauty and noting changes that take place week by week. But in addition, I love the New York metropolitan region for its historical associations. Up in Harriman State Park, for instance, which was a hotbed of activity during the American Revolution, there are ridges and fortifications I like to visit. Sometimes I come across mines. . . . When I'm out hiking, I feel not only part of a natural process, but of a historical one as well."

The relaxation response. That's what walking is all about. In mental terms walking is one of the easiest conceivable ways to back away from stress. Stress is a vital part of the creative process and of achievement, but if unrelieved it can be a major factor in the development of heart disease (as we will see more clearly in later chapters). The body's reaction to stress has been popularly labeled the "fight-or-flight" response. Blood pressure, heart rate, rate of breathing, blood flow to the muscles – all increase in a stressful situation, preparing the body either for conflict or escape. Most of the time, however, we can neither fight nor flee. In business and in family life we lack a natural way to bring the bodily response back to normal again.

There *are* ways to get rid of the tensions. Sport is one way – a violent release that is a socially acceptable alternative to fighting or fleeing. But the violence is not necessary. As Herbert Benson has pointed out in *The Relaxation Response*, it is possible to relax consciously in meditation. The benefits of meditation have now been well researched. Medical analysis of the body's response to transcendental meditation, for instance, has shown that during meditation alpha waves – certain electrical wave patterns in the brain associated with sleep and relaxation – strengthen. Numerous other relaxation techniques elicit the same physical response.

I suggest that walking creates the same liberating effect as sport and meditation, except that it does it better. It does not demand special equipment or the involvement of others or a high level of fitness. Nor does it demand the development of techniques of concentration. The effect is created automatically by movement. Walking irons away anger and tension. After a few minutes, the body imposes its own breathing rhythms, which are not dissimilar to those advocated by yogis. And there are numerous physical benefits – the heart rate increases (rather than declines, as it does in meditation), as does the flow of blood through the veins and arteries. Tension is literally washed away. As the historian George Trevelyan once said,

"I never knew a man go for an honest day's walk for whatever distance, great or small, and not have his reward in the repossession of his soul."

The Tie that Binds

These benefits – and other physical ones which I'll be detailing in later chapters – are yours if you walk, whether you walk in the city or the country, whether you walk alone or with others. Where you walk and who you walk with depends on your personality. I don't mind whether I'm with somebody else or on my own. If in company, I'm happy to talk; but I'm equally happy to wander along in silence. One of the great attractions of walking is that even when you're with somebody, you don't *have* to talk. The slowly changing scenery removes the need for idle chatter. I'm also quite happy to stride out alone, watching or thinking. Or muttering to myself in lonely eccentricity. Walking provides a perfect opportunity to dramatize your tensions away by declaiming brilliantly under your breath as you stride out, rehearsing to yourself the countless scathing or witty remarks that you could have addressed yesterday to boss, spouse, lover, friend or teenage child.

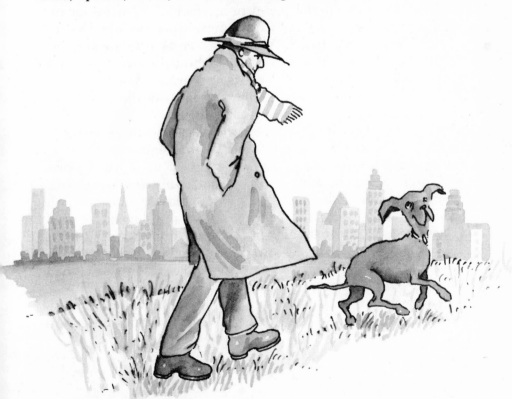

The question of whether to go by yourself or in company has always been a subject of considerable controversy. The English essayist William Hazlitt was a classic loner. "I like to go by myself," he wrote in "Going on a Journey." "I can enjoy society in a room, but out of doors, nature is company enough for me. I am then never less alone than when alone. . . . I cannot see the wit of walking and talking at the same time. . . . The soul of a journey is liberty, perfect liberty to think, feel, do just as one pleases. Give me the clear blue sky over my head, and the green turf beneath my feet, a winding road before me and a three hours' march to dinner – and then to thinking. . . . In company you cannot read the book of nature without being perpetually put to the trouble of translating it for the benefit of others. . . . I like to have it all my own way, and this is impossible unless you are alone." Robert Louis Stevenson agreed: "Freedom is of the essence, because you should be able to stop and go on and follow this way or that as the freak takes you. . . . There should be no cackle of voices at your elbow to jar on the meditative silence of the morning." Sir Max Beerbohm, the suave and scathing English author and caricaturist, argued that walking with a friend inhibited thought and was an excellent way of destroying a friendship (see p. 23).

Yet there is a special pleasure in company, not necessarily the pleasure to be derived from conversation but the pleasure of an experience shared. You may not be able to put your finger on why it is, but each walk can be a unique contribution to a relationship.

Walking is special. Almost all other occasions impose a rigid social framework. A meeting, an office talk, a train ride, a lunch, a drink, a meal with the family – all demand certain reactions that tend to formalize and stylize relationships. But a walk removes the formality. Talk, such as it is, becomes natural, and even small talk – whatever Max Beerbohm's feelings on the subject – seems less small. A remark on the weather becomes a real comment, not simply a social amenity. The silences are not silences at all; they are filled with the pad of feet or the swish of leaves, the sight of scudding clouds or reflected sun. After an hour's walk you will find that you have said less yet feel more at ease with a companion than after an hour spent in almost any other activity. It is the sharing that counts. "Discussions are artificial things, and for the arti-

The Walker as Dullard

Max Beerbohm, the English satirist, takes a jaundiced view of the supposed delights of walking in company.

Walking for walking's sake may be as highly laudable and exemplary a thing as it is held to be by those who practise it. My objection to it is that it stops the brain. Many a man has professed to me that his brain never works so well as when he is swinging along the high road or over hill and dale. This boast is not confirmed by my memory of anybody who on a Sunday morning has forced me to partake of his adventure. Experience teaches me that whatever a fellow-guest may have of power to instruct or to amuse when he is sitting on a chair, or standing on a hearth-rug, quickly leaves him when he takes one out for a walk. The ideas that came so thick and fast to him in any room, where are they now? where that encyclopaedic knowledge which he bore so lightly? where the kindling fancy that played like summer lightning over any topic that was started? The man's face that was so mobile is set now; gone is the light from his fine eyes. He says that A. (our host) is a thoroughly good fellow. Fifty yards further on, he adds that A. is one of the best fellows he has ever met. We tramp another furlong or so, and he says that Mrs. A. is a charming woman. Presently he adds that she is one of the most charming women he has ever known. We pass an inn. He reads vapidly aloud to me: "The King's Arms. Licensed to sell Ales and Spirits." I foresee that during the rest of the walk he will read aloud any inscription that occurs. We pass an "Uxminster. 11 Miles." We turn a sharp corner at the foot of a hill. He points at the wall, and says "Drive Slowly." I see far ahead, on the other side of the hedge bordering the high road, a small notice-board. He sees it too. He keeps his eye on it. And in due course "Trespassers," he says, "Will Be Prosecuted." Poor man! — mentally a wreck.

Luncheon at the A.'s, however, salves him and floats him in full sail. Behold him once more the life and soul of the party. Surely he will never, after the bitter lesson of this morning, go out for another walk. An hour later, I see him striding forth, with a new companion. I watch him out of sight. I know what he is saying. He is saying that I am rather a dull man to go a walk with. He will presently add that I am one of the dullest men he ever went a walk with. Then he will devote himself to reading out the inscriptions.

"You will generally fare better to take your dog than to invite your neighbor. Your cur-dog is a true pedestrian, and your neighbor is very likely a small politician."

John Burroughs, *The Exhilarations of the Road*

---

ficiality of indoors," said philosopher and walking enthusiast C.E.M. Joad, "it's a poor compliment to Nature to use her as an arena for the airing of our views; we do better to let her air our brains."

Who makes good company? The family does – or at least they can do, if you're prepared to accept that family expeditions are *always* fraught with the possibility of unexpected disaster. Children often think they would much rather watch TV than go for a walk. But what do they know? *You* know they'll enjoy themselves once they get out and about, so don't let them miss the opportunity. Suggest, cajole, order them into the right clothing, and drum them out of the house to experience the exhilaration of woods and fields. The ideal, I must admit, is hard to achieve untarnished. Perhaps you have to pile into a car to get anywhere where it's safe to walk. If it's wet, you may find yourself knee-deep in a morass of coats and boots, skirmishing over insoluble problems like missing buttons, sticking zippers, boots with holes, boots that are too large or too small or simply plain uncomfortable ("Don't be silly, darling, of *course* it's not uncomfortable, PUT IT ON!"). In the winter gloves vanish with a facility and regularity that would baffle the most hardened psychic investigator.

Sometimes – if you're like my wife and I – it is simply not worth the trouble. A fractious three-year-old is not good company. How many times have I had a miserable child sitting on my aching shoulders, blinded by tiny fingers grasping for security at my eyelids? How many hours have we spent wrestling in mud with a recalcitrant stroller? And yet we still go on walks, because most of the time we're right: they *do* enjoy it. They explore, they get lost, they get found, they track each other, they climb trees, they do what children are supposed to do on walks. Sometimes it's not even necessary to carry the youngest. I have adopted a trick from my father, who has a simple way of avoiding such burdens. Confronted by the forbidding request "I'm tired, carry me," he replies: "So am I. Let's stand/sit/lie until we're better."

There are times – particularly during a family crisis – when a family walk is the best thing in the world. The intensity of family relationships is often such that in times of crisis rational discussion becomes impossible. A change of job, a new house, problems at school, a driving accident, a daughter's unfortunate choice of boyfriend – all these can bring to the surface tensions and antagonisms that seek to find immediate expression and kill the chance of balanced talk (and also, incidentally, wound relationships that are fundamentally secure). In such circumstances a walk can be as beneficial to a group as it can be to an individual. It is hard to have an argument, let alone sustain one, while walking. The changing sights and sounds, the shifting pattern of links between the members of the group, tend to iron away the petty and the insignificant.

I was once with a family that was having to deal with just such a crisis. Their 17-year-old son had got a 16-year-old girl pregnant. The boy confided in one of the masters at his boarding school. The master took the problem to the headmaster, who was outraged and expelled the boy. The family was appalled by the triple tragedy – the pregnancy and the circumstances which had led to it; the betrayal of trust by the teacher; and the inhumanity of the headmaster. I accompanied them on a walk through a forest after days of endless recrimination. For two hours parents and children mixed and mingled, going over in different ways the various possibilities. By the end of the walk, there was a plan of action. The girl's parents would be invited to talk. Their decision and the daughter's decision about the child would be followed. Financial arrangements would be made. There were other schools for the boy. There were friends he could stay with, subjects he was keen to study. Out of emotional chaos, there arose realistic concern and the beginnings of well-laid plans for practical solutions. (The girl had her baby and is now happily married. The boy went through college and is now a teacher.)

Another way in which company and walking go together is in business. Conferences around a table are fine and I would not suggest a better setting for formalizing arrangements, taking minutes or making set speeches. But often conferences are largely taken up with discussions of complex points that either overwhelm the participants with boredom or else demand a lot of interraction for their solution. One end of the table cannot speak to the other without shouting. Lines of contact all too often become paths for the direction of aggression, and the words weave a web that throbs with tension.

It's seldom done, but in such circumstances breaking up a conference with walking meetings could cut through the boredom and tensions. A group does not walk as a single body. It flows. Links are made, broken and reformed randomly, until one or two assume special significance. If and when they do, groups may form within groups and conversations can explore their own themes without interrupting each other. A walking meeting is a creative process, a simplified image of the brain at work, with cells exchanging information until particular concepts and arguments are well enough formed to bear expression around the conference table.

All around the Town

If you're off for a walk, with or without other people, environment and weather are prime considerations. Town or country, summer or winter, rain or fine, hot or cold – you can experience them all in the course of a few months, and all offer their own interests.

Other chapters cover various aspects of walking in the country – backpacking, nature walking, problems of access – so, before we get into all that, let me say a word about city walking.

It's an underrated and neglected art, yet for a business person or a citybound family it may be your only outlet for walking – and perhaps your only outlet for exercise – for months on end.

Samuel Johnson once said, "The man who is tired of London is tired of life." The same is true of almost any big city you may care to mention. Walking is the only way to feel the pulse of a city and know its character, its vigor, variety and beauty. You may get to know your way around by car or bus, but you can only truly feel the place on foot.

Last summer, while in New York, I found myself walking down 5th Avenue, along Central Park, and decided to record some of my impressions. Starting just above 72nd Street, I was struck by the variety of architecture in this exclusive and re-

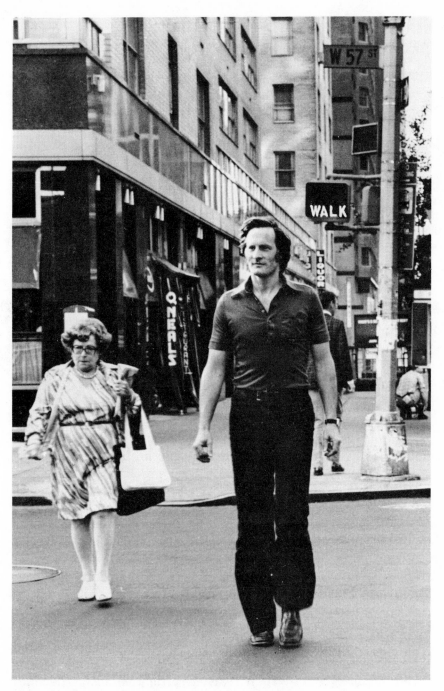

Walking along New York City's 6th Avenue, sensing the human pulse of a supposedly impersonal city.

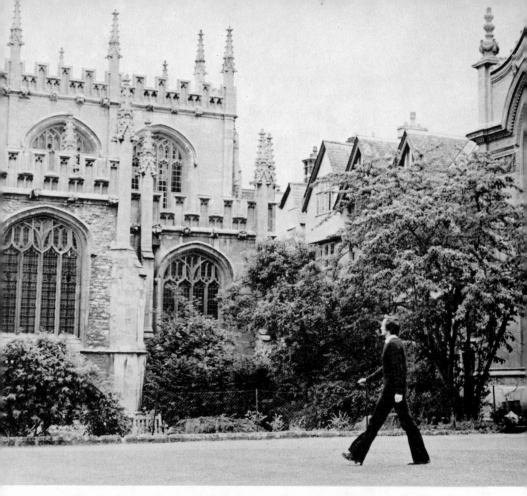

City walking of another kind: past the honeyed stones of Oxford's Brasenose College (right) and St. Mary's Church.

fined area – I'd never bothered to think about it before. I learned later that development in the Upper East Side had only begun when work finished on Central Park itself in 1863; the area's final transformation from open fields to city came in 1907 when the open steam railway along Park Avenue was roofed over. Here, in just half a mile, you can see a cross section of New York's architecture, from the highly decorated, bay-fronted, individual Victorian residences to modern high-rise apartment blocks.

A truck, elaborately decorated with nineteenth-century lettering stood sentinel by some roadworks. Bevies of school-children supervised by their teachers straggled down the side-walk toward the playgrounds and zoo. On my left a low, clas-sically graceful gray building drew my attention. Set behind black railings, it had a beautifully manicured lawn with tulips along the front. It housed the Frick art collection and was designed, I later discovered, by the architects Carrère and Hastings, who also designed the New York Public Library. Opposite was a little classical alcove dedicated to a Richard Morris Hunt: "In recognition of his services to the cause of art in America." (You get to learn how abysmally ignorant you are on walks like these: I had never heard of him, but Hunt was one of America's great architects in the so-called Neo-American Classical of the late nineteenth century and was responsible for the central, pillored pavilion of the Metropolitan Museum of Art.) Scrawled over the inscription in spray paint was a touch of Neo-American Classical of the twentieth century: "Chris SUCKS Nick." (To be fair to both Chris and Nick, someone else had added the middle word.) Nick's signature appeared again on the wall of Central Park, which ran along four foot high on my right. Another bit of graffiti read: "ANDEOTTI = MORO" with the sign of the Red Brigade underneath it, a misspelled reference to the kidnapped (and subsequently murdered) Italian politician Aldo Moro and the current president, Andreotti. On my right was a statue to the 7th Regiment New York, 107th United States Infantry, an *in memoriam* for the First World War – a powerful work in metal I had never noticed before.

At 63rd Street on a park bench a young smartly turned-out black sat with an enormous radio turned up full blast. A little beyond stood two small stalls of books set up by Barnes & Noble. The stall holder told me they have to rent the space from the city. "It doesn't make any money. We do it for advertising purposes." A few yards further and I was almost at the southern-most end of the park. I suddenly found myself amidst hot-dog stands and soft-drink sellers. In front of me was the Plaza Hotel, its sixteen stories capped by its steep, chateau-style roof.

A mere thirteen blocks, but it was enough to show me that with senses properly tuned, one can sop up a good deal of a city's life. But there's more to a city than sights, sounds and a

---

"To enjoy city walking to the utmost you have to throw yourself into a mood of loving humanity."

Donald Culross Peattie, *The Joy of Walking*

"You can't get the best of a city from a taxi or a bus (to say nothing of a subway) . . . you learn a city only by walking it."
Joseph Wood Krutch, *Is Walking the New Status Symbol?*

---

bit of history. It's possible to look still deeper and see them as expressions of the natural world made of materials put together from countless different areas. Nature may be suppressed in a city, but it is not totally extinguished.

Beneath an arch that leads into the Natural History Museum in New York is a stalactite. Water has seeped through the rock – granite about two billion years old from the shores of the St. Lawrence – dissolved the cement and redeposited it, as if in a cave, in an upsidedown pillar. In the cracks in the museum steps, mosses and small plants flourish. Over the years water has entered the cracks, frozen and expanded, shrugging the block of granite out of true and allowing space for soil and seeds to gather.

Such processes show nature at work in the heart of a city. It's a study that is of special interest to one of the museum geologists, Sid Horenstein, who runs nature tours in the heart of Manhattan. A walk around the city with him puts things in a totally new light. "Look at the ginko tree," he will say, "a living fossil. Before the eighteenth century, it was only found in and around Chinese and Japanese shrines. The trees would be extinct now if they hadn't been preserved. The first European to see one was a doctor attached to the Dutch East India Company, when he visited Nagasaki in 1690. Over the millennia, it has become extraordinarily resistant. It was introduced over here in the 1800s and doesn't seem to be affected by the city's pollution."

"Now, look here," he'll say suddenly, pointing to some faint scrawling marks in the rock from which a high-rise building is made. "Worm casts. This building is full of fossils. See here? Shells, snails, corals. Tiny, but still fossils. This stone came from Indiana. A hundred million years ago it was at the bottom of a shallow sea. That's when these fossils were deposited."

With Sid by your side, walking in the city is like being in a mobile paleontology lab. He's even planning a tour called "The Fossils of 42nd Street." On one of the many walks we took last

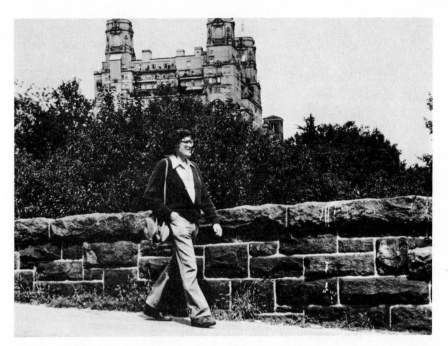

City naturalist Sid Horenstein strolling into Central Park.

year, we strolled into the lobby of an old apartment building, a lavish marble-and-stone interior from the late nineteenth century. It turned out to be a geological museum in miniature. "Here are sections of oysters from Trieste. They're in a limestone about eighty million years old. Here's some travertine from Italy. See all these holes? That's where mosses used to live. The Colosseum is built of stones like this. This purplish-bluey rock is Tennessee Marble."

Outside, the street turned into a veritable valley of natural wonder. "The starlings up there are not natural to New York City. Forty pairs were released in Central Park in the 1890s. Now they range across the entire US, northern Mexico and southern Canada –"

"Look at the grasses around this drain, six, seven species –"

"See the way the lamp post bends over at the top? See the hole? Birds nest in there –"

"You can never be bored walking in New York, or in any city, you know. Irrespective of the people and the variety of the architecture, there's so much to see and know about once you wake up to it. The stones, the plants, the animals, even water

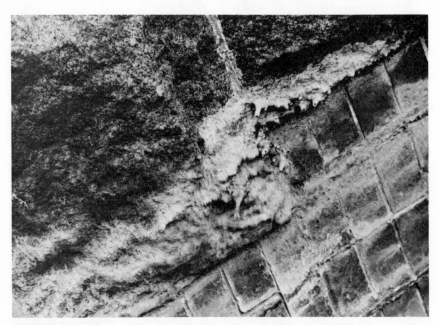

Stalactites beneath an arch, flanking the American Museum of Natural History.

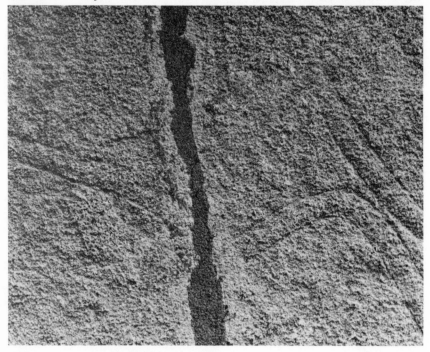

Fossil wormcasts in a stone facade.

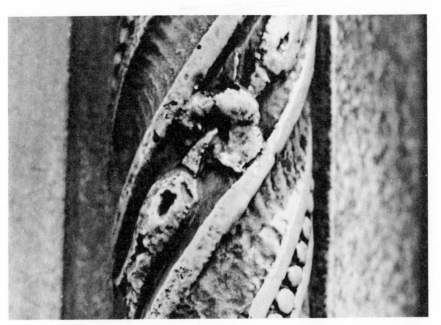

Travertine marble from Italy in a nineteenth-century apartment lobby.

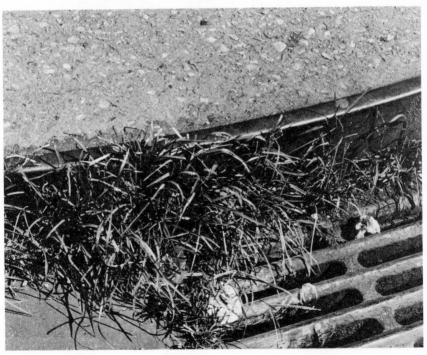

A habitat in miniature: several species of grass crowd a drain.

33

gushing from a hydrant, like a spring, all remind me that the city is not an unnatural place at all, but just a special sort of natural place."

Whatever the Weather

Finally, what weather makes the best walking? Most people would say a warm, summer's day which demands no equipment and offers lush, picture-postcard views. The delights of such days are obvious, and I won't dwell on them. Let me instead put forward two alternatives – for winter walking and for walking in the rain.

Winter is glorious for walking if, like me, you don't mind the damp. If there is ice and a sprinkling of snow, so much the better. It's both secure and exhilarating to feel the tang of cold air, the unaccustomed rigidity of frozen mud or the swish of frost-encrusted grass. As the walking philosopher C.E.M. Joad says: "In the winter I can go across country. There is no undergrowth in the woods; there are no crops in the fields and no bracken on the slopes. One walks free and unencumbered and, broadly speaking, one walks where one likes.

"And how much one sees! In August the country is muffled under a blanket of dull green. The blanket spoils its shape and blots its contours. The winds of winter have stripped the blanket away and laid bare the bones and naked structure of the countryside. And how lovely that structure is! I would give all the tender greens of young spring, all the gorgeous colors of autumn woods' decay, for the bare boughs of an oak with its tracery of little twigs silhouetted against the dark red of an afternoon sky in December. The sun has just set and over against it, glimpsed through the infinitely lovely pattern work of the twigs, there is an evening star. There is a tang in the air; the earth rings hard under the feet; there will be a frost to-

---

"I find a charm in rainy prospects; the dull colours are more velvety, the flat tones grow more tender. The landscape is like a face that has been weeping; it is less beautiful, certainly, but more expressive."

Henri Frederic Amiel, *What a Lovely Walk*!

---

night. What has summer to offer comparable to these winter delights?''

And what of the joys of rain? True, being caught in a rainstorm unsuitably prepared is a misery. Nobody wants to be soaked through and cold. But there are exceptions. I was once caught in a hot summer downpour along with an army of children during a picnic beside the Thames. We were two miles from home when thunder clouds rolled up out of nowhere. "OK, kids, be warned," I shouted, "you're going to get wet, enjoy it!" When the rain came, we did, all the way home. Like walking in winter, walking in the rain – light rain, when you're suitably clad – is a pleasure all its own. Summer rain refreshes and reassures. Winter rain invigorates. The weather is never as bad outside as it looks from within.

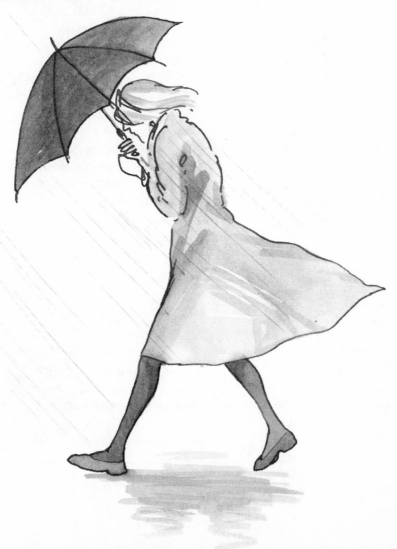

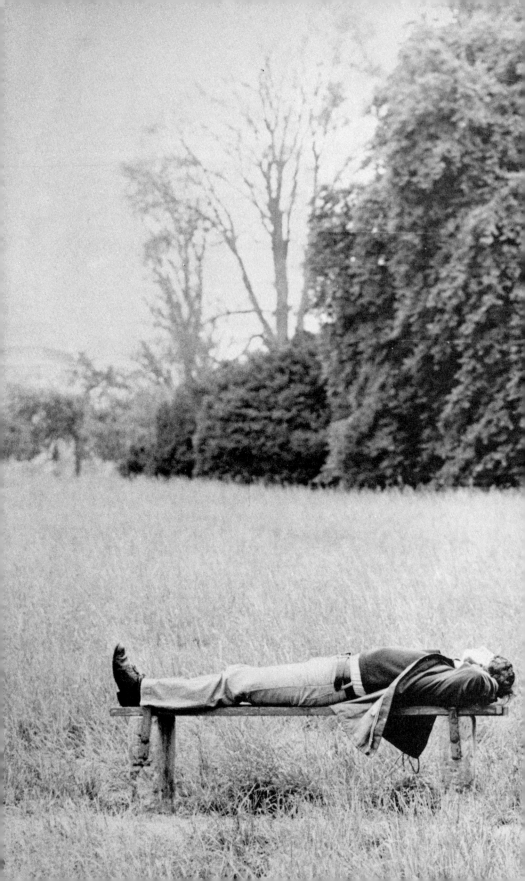

Why Not Walk Before You Run?

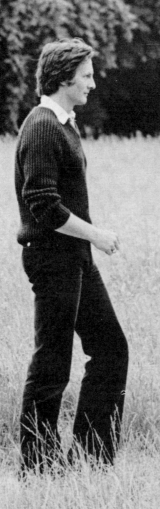

Why Not Walk
Before You Run?

WHY WALK? Because it makes you feel good and makes you look good. That is, of course, the same thing that runners claim. So, as long as you're basically fit, why not get out there and head toward fitness as fast as you can with a full-fledged, hard-breathing, hard-sweating exercise program?

Good question. I decided to find out the answer by speaking to the "Guru of Runners" (the epithet is now almost synonomous with his name) – Dr. George Sheehan. I somehow expected him to advocate running as the be-all and end-all for a fit and happy life. Not so at all.

"I think jogging is completely unnecessary for a fitness program," he said categorically. "A good brisk walk is equivalent to a jog anytime."

We weren't, of course, talking about the super-fit, but about those who were beginning to exercise after many years of sloth. "No, I would never recommend jogging to patients who are relatively unfit people," Dr. Sheehan went on. "I say, well, you have to go for thirty minutes a day, and you can walk it in the beginning. You should start at a pace at which you can talk with someone. If you're unused to exercise, you can't possibly do that at a jog."

In fact the running boom has, in some ways, made his task more difficult. Walking is such a natural activity that people tend to ignore its beneficial potential. "When people come to me to ask about exercise," said Dr. Sheehan, "many of them have the feeling inside that they should be doing more. I try to disabuse them of that. Jogging is a more psychological necessity than a physical one."

I then asked him the obvious question: "But if you don't necessarily recommend running for other people, why do you do it yourself?"

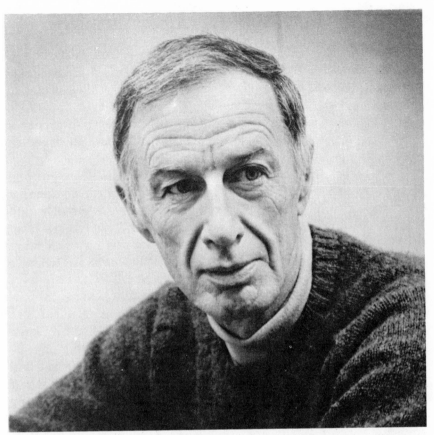

Although the author of the best-selling Running and Being, *Dr. George Sheehan is no doctrinaire advocate of running. He advises walking both for beginners and for those fit enough to run who don't enjoy running for its own sake.*

"Oh, I do it for my own reasons," he replied. "I don't presume to know what happens with anybody else. I like to get into my own head and I like to escape from the environment. If you get much above 5 MPH, you begin to lose sense impressions. It's my own form of relaxation, a combination of East and West, of meditation and sweating – the best of both worlds if you like. But it's not for everybody."

Nor should it be. It takes years for anyone to build up to Sheehan's level of fitness, and it takes many hours a week – some of them very painful hours – to stay there. For us ordinary mortals, walking is the best way to start, and often as good a way as any to continue.

Looking the Revolution Straight in the Eye

It has been estimated that there are in the United States some ten to fifteen million joggers (or runners, as they now prefer to call themselves). The percentage is lower in Britain, but there must be over a million of them and the number is noticeably increasing week after week, as it is throughout the western world.

Now, there are many good things to be said for running. Physically and mentally it can lead to a richer life, and does for tens of thousands of people. But there are many ways in which it is demanding, painful and even dangerous (as we'll see later on in this chapter). There is, however, something even more worrying about the running revolution: What of those who are *not* touched by it?

There are millions of people who have neither the time nor the inclination – not to mention the basic fitness needed – to confront the challenge of running. I have talked to many such nonrunners and found two related reactions among them.

Firstly, there are those who feel vaguely criticized and put down by the hordes who pound the concrete outside their doors. There is a strong implication in the literature of running that runners are not only physically superior, but spiritually superior as well. In the first issue of a new weekly, *On the Run*, editor and publisher Bob Anderson states categorically that his religion is "runner." It gives him, he says, both spiritual and physical health. "I have found through running that I became the power and the light." This seems an unfortunate judgment on those who are not of the Elect, and do not want to be.

Secondly, there are those among the non-Elect, many millions of people throughout the western world, who are excluded simply because they are genuinely unfit, and know it. They

---

"All walking is discovery. On foot we take the time to see things whole. We see trees as well as forests, people as well as crowds."

Hal Borland, *To Own the Streets and Fields*

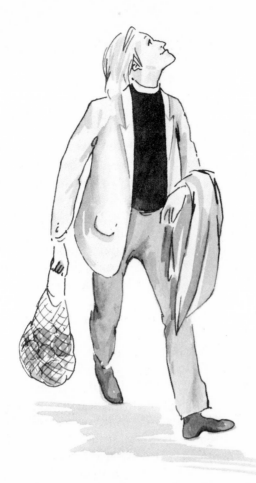

work hard, they drink, they smoke, they enjoy their food, they are overweight. They take little or no exercise. We all know them . . . husbands and fathers who are beginning to worry about their hearts and wonder if they should be changing their life styles; thick-waisted and heavy-thighed wives and mothers who diet occasionally, only to find the regimen tough to take and the results all too brief. For such people, change is hard. However important they know it is to cut out cigarettes, to cut down on alcohol, to lose weight, to take exercise, they don't know how to begin. It's no good telling them to get out and run. The suggestion merely points out inadequacies they already know. They feel threatened and criticized, and their reaction is a very human one: they withdraw from the problem.

A friend of mine, Dr. Ian Anderson, who runs a heart clinic in London, has had direct experience of this. "The people who

I see regularly are usually highly motivated individuals who intend to do something about their life," he says, "but what about the others? They are frightened of confronting their own deficiencies." He went on to tell me about his attempt to interest a large advertising company in setting up a preventive medical program. The chairman arrived for an exercise test, and the benefits of combining a small amount of exercise with a more controlled life style were explained to him. "Tell me about your board members," Ian had asked him. "What kind of shape are they in?" Predictably, all eight board members smoked and were overweight; all were under 50. A carefully controlled program of exercise and dieting would certainly improve their health, Ian explained, and it could be paid for from tax-deductible sources. The personal and corporate benefits would be immense. The chairman agreed that it would be a good idea for his whole board to come along and have a test. "But not one of them was prepared to come," Ian told me. "They just didn't want to know."

At the Heart of the Matter

Attitudes like this are understandable to a certain extent, but they can also be fatal. The message of this chapter is a simple one: No one needs to feel put down for refusing to join the running revolution. Nor does anyone need to feel threatened by it. The point is that it is perfectly possible to confront the physical problems that beset almost everyone as they approach and go beyond middle age without the sudden and dramatic change of life style that running so often demands. The secret is to take it slowly and naturally and enjoy what you do – by walking, for starters. With that as your foundation, you can be fit for anything.

But before I suggest some answers, let's review the problems to emphasize that there is a need to build *some* physical activity into your life. Of the two million deaths every year in the United States, about half are caused by failures of the cardiovascular system. Among American males between the ages of 33 and 65 – the most productive years, when a man is doing most for his family and society – coronary heart disease causes one-third of the deaths – about 250,000 each year. For every death, there is another nonfatal attack, each spreading its ripples of shock and fear among family and friends. Heart and blood vessel diseases cost the United States an estimated $28.5 billion each year and the loss of an estimated 52 million days of production. Britain is slightly better off – some 150,000 deaths are caused by coronary heart disease each year and the country loses about 7 million working days – but the figures are rising faster in Britain than in the United States (where they have, over the past few years, actually shown a slight but reassuring drop).

Coronary heart disease is largely the result of atherosclerosis, a condition in which the linings of the arteries become progressively thickened by deposits of fat and other chemical debris. Gradually the arteries lose their pliability and become narrower, restricting normal blood flow. When one of the vessels that supplies the heart becomes blocked, a heart attack results. The part of the heart muscle supplied by the blocked artery fails to receive sufficient oxygen and other nutrients and begins to die. It is a process that begins early. A famous study of Korean War combat casualties showed that 70 percent had coronary atherosclerosis in some form – yet the average age of those studied was just over 22.

Coronary heart disease is the major killer in western civilization. Its vast incidence seems to be an unprecedented phenomenon, related to habits imposed on us by the society in which we live – a largely sedentary existence with liberal supplies of good food and drink, and ready access to tobacco. Identifying the various factors involved and assessing the significance of each is at present the subject of intensive research.

It is generally agreed among researchers that no one factor is sufficient to explain the high incidence of coronary heart disease in the West today. A number of factors have been identified, however, and there is not much anyone can do about some of them: statistically, an individual is more at risk if there is a history of heart disease in the family; if he is a man; if he is white; and if he is over 65. But there are other contributing factors that are under individual control, at least in theory. In summary these are:

1. High blood pressure: Blood pressure is a measure of the force the heart must exert to push blood through the veins and arteries. The more clogged they are, the higher the pressure required and the greater the risk. A man whose blood pressure at systole (the moment the heart contracts) is over 150 has more than twice the risk of a heart attack and nearly four times the risk of a stroke than a man whose systolic blood pressure is under 120.

2. Cigarettes: Coronary attacks are three times as common in moderate smokers (fifteen cigarettes a day) as in nonsmokers under the age of 55, and the risk of sudden death is five times as great. Men aged 40 to 49 who smoke forty cigarettes a day have five times the risk of dying from coronary heart disease as non-smokers. About 95 percent of patients with arterial disease are smokers. Professor D.D. Reid of the London School of Hygiene has calculated that of every hundred deaths attributable to heavy smoking about sixteen may be due to lung cancer, but no fewer than fifty may result from coronary heart disease.

3. Cholesterol: The fatty deposits in arteries consist largely of cholesterol, a complex, crystalline alcohol that is one of the most common substances in the body. The amount of cholesterol in the blood varies widely. Cholesterol comes from two sources – the body makes its own and it is taken in as part of any diet that includes animal fats. Most men in western society have a cholesterol level in the range of 130–260 milligrams per 100 milliliters of blood. A man with a blood cholesterol measurement of 250 milligrams or more has about three times the risk of having a heart attack or stroke as a man with a blood cholesterol reading of 94 milligrams.

4. Obesity: After the age of 25 the average individual tends to gain a pound of weight per year or ten pounds every decade if food intake remains the same. In other words, the eating habits of youth are inappropriate to middle age. At the same time, each one of us tends to lose one-quarter to one-half of a pound of fat-free weight (muscle, bone, skin, etc.) each year. By 55, therefore, the average individual, unless he or she does something about it, can end up a good forty pounds overweight, with consequences that do more than simply overburden the heart. The extra weight, simply as a result of the mechanical problems it brings, increases the risk of arthritis, joint trouble (especially in the hips and knees), flat feet and varicose veins.

The Fate of Homo Sedentarius

*The general physiological effect of the Western life style is graphically
summarized by Dr. Henry Blackburn:*

Modern man in industrial society is an animal which, shortly
after maturation, is confined to a system of special cages, in
one of which, a mobile steel and plastic cage, he is exposed for
one or two hours daily to complex decisions, frustration and
danger, in an atmosphere high in carbon-monoxide, while
transported to and from other cages. In these other cages,
under constant temperature environments, the animal's
physical activity is strictly constrained to many hours of sitting
and a few moments daily of standing, with short, level walks,
all of very low-energy expenditure. The industrialized species
of man is habitually overfed with animal and grain chow which
usually includes 20 percent of all calories from saturated fats,
20 percent from refined carbohydrates, and 10 percent from
fermented spirits, plus varying concentrations of herbicides,
pesticides, hormones, antibiotics, oxidizing agents, and radio-
active isotopes. Man is systematically conditioned to self-
administer twenty potent doses of nicotine, and five of caffeine
alkaloids daily. He is also trained to lie motionless in a darkened
cage for three hours and watch a cathode ray tube which
continuously presents ambiguous information and repeated
suggestions for unhygienic, purposeless activity. He is rewarded to the degree that he pursues this goal-less activity
during the day.
Exposed to such an environment for half his life span,
nearly all the animals develop largely irreparable lesions in the
vascular system, and about half of the male animals experience
severe damage to cardiac muscle.

5. **Stress:** Anger, fear, irritation and excitement, all prepare
the body for vigorous muscular action by speeding up the heart
and releasing fats and sugars into the bloodstream for use as
instant energy. This is usually known as the "fight-or-flight"
response. The ambitious executive confronted by an office crisis
only occasionally indulges in extreme physical activity – and
even then, it's usually inappropriate to the body's needs (I know
of one newspaper executive who regularly throws his telephone
through a closed window in times of stress).

So Much for Sedentary Living

And so much for the bad news. You can see exactly how bad it is by assessing your own risk of a heart attack in the next chapter (p. 62) and Appendix 1 at the back of the book. The good news is that the most serious problem areas which I've listed above can be controlled. Regular, long-term training – the kind provided by a basic walking program, which I'll outline in later chapters – can have a marvelous effect. The heart can increase up to 15 percent in size. It can be made to pump slower and more powerfully under stress. The trained heart speeds up less, yet pumps out more – thirty to thirty-six liters a minute in an athlete compared with twenty-four liters a minute in a sedentary person. Moreover, the trained body can extract more oxygen from the blood and deal with fats more efficiently.

There is a classic case study conducted by Professor J.N. Morris and his colleagues of the Medical Research Council's Social Medicine Research Unit in London in 1953 that effectively demonstrates the beneficial results of exercise. They compared the number of coronary heart disease cases in a large group of drivers of double-decker London buses with the number of cases found among the conductors (ticket collectors), whose jobs were more active. Morris and his colleagues found that the conductors, bounding up and down stairs for several hours a day, suffered fatal heart attacks at only half the rate of their highly stressed, sedentary colleagues.

True, Morris and his team also found that the drivers were less active and less generally fit to begin with (the trousers the drivers were issued when they joined the bus service averaged at least an inch more round the waist than the conductors' trousers), but the results are still hard to ignore.

Other follow-up studies have supported the obvious conclusion. Among male American railroad employees the annual death rate from coronary heart disease has been found to be 7.6 percent for laborers and 11.8 percent for clerks. In a study of hospitalized coronary patients, the death rate in the first month was 8.2 percent for heavy workers, but 18.8 percent for light workers.

From 1968 to 1970 Morris and his group assessed almost 17,000 male sedentary civil servants. By the end of September 1972, 232 men had suffered some sort of attack. Their life styles

---

"He was about 10 years old, sandy-haired, stocky, deeply tanned . . . I quickened my step and caught up with him . . . I asked, 'Just why are you walking them?'

He became very serious. 'To get tough,' he said. 'I want to be quarterback on our team, and I got to get tough.'"

Hal Borland, *To Own the Streets and Fields*

---

were compared with those who had not suffered attacks. It turned out that only 23 of the coronary victims were exercisers; the rest were sedentary. Conversely, heavy exercisers did *not* suffer their fair share of coronaries. Among the activities that seemed to offer some protection were hill climbing, brisk walking in town or over rough country, and climbing over five hundred stairs daily (which sounds like a lot, but is equivalent to no more than the three or four flights an hour done by many office workers who do not rely on elevators to get them where they're going). One interesting finding from this study was that brisk activity apparently also offered some protection from the risks of cigarette smoking. In men taking vigorous exercise, the relative risks were 36 percent of average for nonsmokers and 50 percent for smokers.

Other studies have tended to confirm these findings. For instance, an analysis of the 55,000 men in the Health Insurance Program of Urban New York shows a dramatic difference in the incidence of heart attack deaths between the "least active" and the "moderately active" groups. The "moderately active" men simply tended to walk a few extra blocks or climb stairs a little more. A study done in Evans County, Georgia, reveals that an expenditure of a mere 400–500 calories per week above average was enough to confer some protection from heart disease. Britain's Geoffrey Rose has reported that walking twenty minutes or more to work was associated with a 30 percent decrease in the incidence of a poor supply of blood to the heart. Longshoremen who increased their calory expenditure by almost 1,000 calories per day reduced the incidence of coronary heart disease among their numbers by 25 percent.

The conclusion of all these studies now seems obvious to many doctors. As Dr. William Kannel stated in *The New England Journal of Medicine:*

Over the years, except for diet, little has been more subject to fadism than physical culture. With the proportion of virtually motionless persons in the general population growing, the need to gain the habit of walking and climbing stairs seems urgent . . . it is time to consider engineering physical activity back into daily living to counter the sloth and gluttony promulgated by modern technology.

Those are the scientific findings. In a way they state the obvious. *Of course* one should keep active. *Of course* one should keep the body doing what it has evolved to do – whether hunting, feeding, attacking or defending. Tribal communities and our own ancestors could only survive by being active and ready for action. Whatever freedoms urban life gives us, it does deprive us of the immediate need for a tough body. It is a need that has to be reasserted if we are to live life to the full.

It is this basic truism that lies, in part, behind the running revolution.

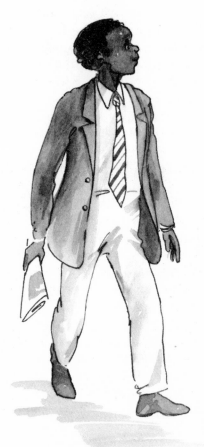

Have You Had Your "Fixx" Today?

Let's look for a moment at this startling phenomenon by ticking off some of the facts about it. James Fixx's *Complete Book of Running* has been a long-"running" bestseller throughout the English-speaking world. In 1977 Americans alone spent $257 million on running equipment. For countless 40-to-50-year-olds, running has become an addiction: they need their daily "Fixx."

"I'd have welcomed a mugger or two," said a 51-year-old runner friend of mine describing an outing he'd taken in Central Park on a recent trip to New York. "There's more danger of being flattened by joggers." The New York Road Runners Club has more than 16,000 members. There are now at least 50,000 Americans who have completed at least one marathon. Catering to them is a new, fat, glossy monthly entitled simply *Marathoner*. During any weekend, almost any medium-sized city stages a race with 500-plus participants. The big marathons – like those in Boston and New York City – attract thousands. Need I go on? No wonder one of the high priests of running, Thaddeus Kostrubala, compares the significance of the running revolution to the impact of the Crusades and the introduction of dental hygiene.

I can see why runners run. An action well done by a body highly tuned gives a feeling of power, of control over oneself, and, in a small way, over one's destiny. Running drives out tensions, it fills leisure time and, once you are fit, it makes you feel good . . .

And yet, and yet. There are millions who will not run and who will never run. It will never make *them* feel good, because they will never do it. To them, running seems a pointless activity. You don't get anywhere, you don't win anything, you risk making a fool of yourself. Another friend, an administrator in a New York school, commented dismissively "All they're doing is breathing in the pollution."

"The walker can find his inner world no more than a short stroll from home. . . . The walker has found the peace that the runner still seeks."

George Sheehan, *Dr. Sheehan on Running*

If that is the way you feel, take heart. Running is not all joy. In fact it can hurt like hell and lead to serious injury. For the dedicated runner, pain is an acceptable part of the regimen. It is the latter-day equivalent of the hair shirt and flagellation, part of a search for physical and spiritual purity. But for the unconverted, a review of the dangers of jogging may bring a certain reassurance.

The Agony of Ecstasy

There is one fearful danger to running, at least for the unfit who seek an instant change in life style: *running can be fatal.*

It is a familiar enough story. Remember so-and-so? Deputy head of finance at the Enormous Sums of Money Corporation. Brilliant career ahead of him. How old was he? Forty-five? Forty-six? Didn't look any older anyway, especially in a business suit. Bit chubby, of course. Smoked a bit. Liked a martini, now and then. Know what happened? Got the fitness bug last weekend. A mile from home, dropped dead in his track suit. Shame really. Nice fellow.

There are no official figures quantifying the deaths from jogging, but every doctor has an anecdote to make the point. And how many times a year does your local newspaper record the death of a family man or business executive indulging in unaccustomed exercise? In June 1978 I made my first visit to Washington while researching this book. I was there for just one day. On the front page of the *Washington Post,* above the headline "Fatality at Protest" were two pictures, one of doctors trying to resuscitate a cardiac victim, David Wilson, 46, a Health, Education and Welfare employee. Another showed his distraught wife, Cynthia. Wilson had collapsed and died at the end of a three-mile jog protesting against HEW's enforcement of a law on sex discrimination in education. A few weeks later in Miami, Robert Summers, the 55-year-old administrator of the Miami Heart Institute, was found dead on a street near his home. He, too, had been out jogging. OK, to be fair it's not just running . . . In 1972 Godfrey Wynn, the famous English broadcaster, died at the age of 62 during a game of tennis. The examples are countless.

Twenty years ago doctors, friends and family would have drawn an obvious but oversimplified conclusion from such occurrences: if you are unfit, don't risk straining your heart by exercising. But given the abundance of findings on the benefits of exercise over the last ten years, the advice must now be: exercise, but exercise with care. If you are unused to physical activity, have a medical checkup; and anyway, whatever your age, start slowly. If you don't, and if you push yourself too hard and too fast, watch out for trouble. (Just *how* you start, we will get to in the next two chapters.)

Even Dr. George Sheehan, America's best-known advocate of running, has had his problems as a middle-aged runner, especially at the beginning. His personal experience should be taken to heart by anybody who is considering taking up running as a quick way to achieve an overall sense of well-being.

"When I took up distance running in my mid-40s, I rewrote my life story," he wrote in one of his popular editorials in *The Physician and Sportsmedicine*. "It has become a biography of pain. I discovered that the middle-aged person is the perfect laboratory animal for research in sports medicine. . . . I was not sleek, quick or instinctive. I was ragged, slow and unco-ordinated, more often limping than not. As time passed. I developed every overused syndrome in the books and some that weren't. Instead of reading about diseases, I got them. I became a mobile medical museum, a clinical exhibit of the illnesses of distance runners."

What are the ailments to which runners are so peculiarly susceptible? Let's start with the bottom line – the foot. The human foot is a remarkable piece of engineering. Its twenty-eight bones combine to fulfill a double role: each foot is a rigid lever when it pushes forward and a flexible cushion that takes up the force of contact when it meets the ground at the end of each stride. The treatment this superbly adaptable device can sustain is staggering. Our feet are built to carry us an average of 65,000 miles, or two-and-a-half times round the earth, in a lifetime. Soccer players in a single game take as many as 10,000 steps, with an accumulated impact per foot of a thousand tons.

Yet the foot is by no means perfect in evolutionary terms (let alone in terms of the peculiar faults that can develop in an individual's lifetime). When I went to see Dr. Richard Schuster of the New York College of Podiatric Medicine about foot problems in walking and running, he pointed out some of our

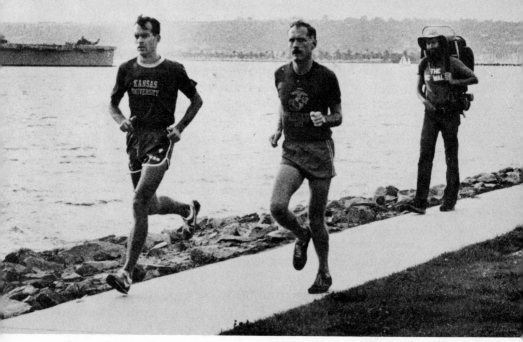

Faster but not fitter: walker Gary Moore gives a self-assured smile as two runners pant past him along San Diego Bay, California.

inherited disadvantages. "Before you're born, you're rolled up into a ball," he explained, "a rather snug ball. The human – of all the primates – has the biggest head. It is also the best bipedal walker of all primates, so in addition it has the longest legs. A human fetus has a big head and long legs – and no place to put them. It's all crouched up, with its legs crossed. Did you know we're the only primate that develops with our legs crossed? While we are crouched up in the uterus, sideways pressure pushes the legs, the heels and the forefeet inwards. Just look at any newborn child: it lies with its feet facing inwards. That's usually outgrown by the age of 7 or 8, but we retain a tendency to invert the feet. It is our body weight that forces them flat."

"I thought evolution would have come to terms with the demands of our life style by now," I remarked.

"No, no, evolution is not a comfortable thing," Dr. Schuster replied. "Twenty-five or thirty million years ago, the foot was not a foot; it was a hand. It had to evolve into a foot as our ancestors descended from the trees. But we still retain the characteristics of that hand. Many people's feet have a big toe that points a bit away from the other toes. Put your hand out in front of you." I did. "You see how the thumb hangs down a little? Some people's toes do that. You can think of hand-like characteristics such as this as evolutionary scars on our feet."

Considering all of which, our feet don't do so badly. In every mile walked, each foot sustains the gravity-induced impact of several thousand pounds without any apparent strain. Our feet can usually take unprotestingly a variety of surfaces, from concrete in badly fitting shoes to a soft sand dune barefoot.

But there are limits. A walker imposes perhaps 120 percent of his body weight on each foot. A runner imposes up to four times that weight. At each pace, a 180-pound runner sprinting on a hard surface slams about 700 pounds through a few square inches of bone and each foot will slap down 5,000 times an hour. Even at a light jog, each foot sustains an accumulated 1,000+ tons in the course of an hour.

For some people, it is just too much. The most common complaints are inflammation of the *plantar fascia* (the tight band of tissue which runs from the toes to the heel), heel bruising, inflamed tendons, blisters, ingrown toenails and nerve damage. Dr. Steve Subotnick, foot specialist, runner and contributor to *Runner's World* magazine, estimates that about half the population have foot bones that are a degree or two out of true. For them, the stress of running thirty-plus miles a week is even more intense.

These are problems that all runners must be prepared to face. For many, they simply become a painful part of everyday life. But for those who are newcomers at trying to get fit, such aches and pains can be a disaster – not so much in physical terms (the treatment is usually simple: rest), but psychologically. A 40-year-old man or woman new to jogging, who comes down with Achilles tendonitis after a couple of days, may have to rest for several weeks before he or she feels strong enough and physically confident to try again. The chances are that such people will *never* try again. They have experienced pain, been temporarily crippled and gained nothing. They'll probably con-

---

"Like Hamlet, I 'throw physic to the dogs,' and let my feet take care of themselves."

A. N. Cooper, *Sore Feet*

---

clude that they may just as well remain unfit without injury.

The foot is just the beginning of a runner's problems. The stresses imposed by running have other effects – on ankles, leg muscles and knees. In the US the most widely discussed injuries are those that go under the general rubric of "shin splints." Runners say they have shin splints if they experience any pain between knee and ankle. I've never been affected, and was puzzled by the term (it's not commonly used in England). Dr. Gil Gleim at the Institute of Sports Medicine and Athletic Trauma at Lenox Hill Hospital in Manhattan, tried to demystify it for me. "It's a catch-all phrase," he said. "As a professor of mine in college used to say, if you don't know what the cause is, put a label on it anyway and everyone will be happy. This particular label applies to tenderness with many causes. If you feel any runner's leg on the inside of the shinbone and press down, he or she is likely to be tender there. I would say that virtually every runner has that tenderness at some time or another."

Doctors have mentioned many causes for shin splints. They include: bad style, a change of running shoe, muscular imbalance, doing too much too quickly, weak arches, and a change in running surface. The results are equally varied, but all painful. Calf muscles are strained, muscle attachments separate from the thin tissue encasing the bones, tendons become inflamed and in extreme cases the bones themselves develop hairline fractures. As yet, no one has pinpointed a direct cause-and-effect progression of this affliction. Treatment is as varied as the possible causes: runners tape themselves up, try strengthening exercises, invest in new pairs of shoes, slap on ice packs, go in for ultrasound and inject Novocain and steroids. But the best treatment of all is: stop running.

Then again, take jogger's knee, in which the cartilage in the knee joint is eroded by stress; Dr. Gleim estimates that "well over 50 percent of runners at one time or another have experienced knee pain." Or take your pick of medial arch strain, chronic subluxation, pronation, Morton's foot syndrome . . .

I won't labor the point further. Instead I'll back off and let Russell Baker, writing in *The New York Times Magazine* in June 1978, have a say. Put off the activity at an early age through a combination of boredom, pain and hopelessness, here he is reminiscing about the bittersweet joys of high school running:

The aim is to achieve a complete physical collapse, just short of death, simultaneously with hitting the finish tape. Not being permitted to die, at least when I was at high school, one was permitted to vomit, after which you jogged a little to "cool off." . . . Why, you will ask, should anyone submit to such torment? . . . What a question. This was high school. . . . Youth is a time of enduring agonies without asking why. I knew that even then. I would endure, I told myself, but when I grew up I would never run again. Or jog. To me, being grown up meant, besides being able to buy beer without having to prove my age, never having to engage in athletics for which I was inadequately constructed.

Baker goes on to suggest that nonjoggers perform an important social role. They provide joggers with a justification for jogging: "Contemplating imminent demise among the sedentary helps the athletic to endure their suffering."

Most of us are not so philanthropic. We know we should keep moving. But why not do it without the risk of injury?

In short, why not try *walking* your way to fitness instead of running there? If you're anything like me, you'll find it an easier, safer, less strenuous and infinitely more enjoyable way of getting there. By following a regular walking program you can, in time, build exactly the same level of fitness that you can with a basic running program . . . and with much less agony and suffering along the way.

Think you're ready? Go on to the next chapter, and let's find out.

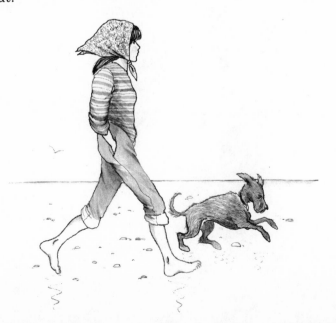

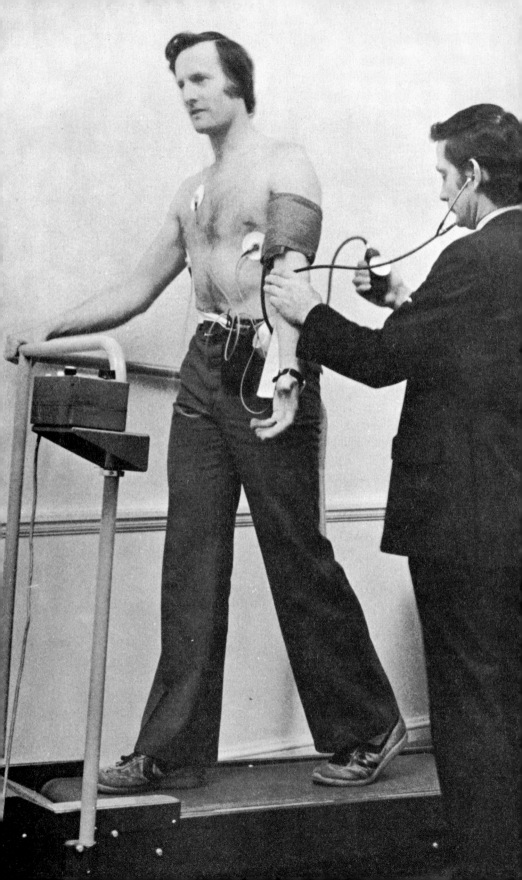

Testing, Testing

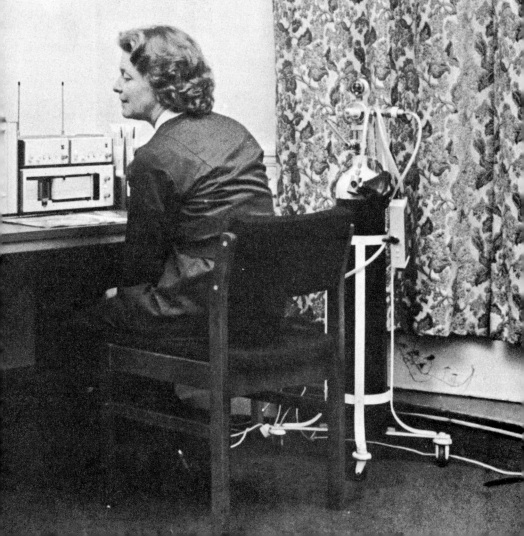

Testing, Testing

B Y FAR THE STRONGEST incentive to undertake a walking
program – or any exercise program, for that matter – is to be
on the receiving end of a heart attack. Countless exhortations
from well-meaning friends and from authors like myself are
like whispers in a storm compared to the brief protest of an
overburdened heart. Many thousands of people have, of
course, suffered a small heart attack, recovered with the aid of
a program of regular exercise which completely changed their
lives, and thus benefited from their brush with catastrophe.
These people apart for a moment (for I'll be dealing with heart
attack victims more fully in the chapter devoted to "Special
Problems"), let's take a closer look at the *second* most powerful
incentive to get moving: the realization of just how generally
unfit you really are.

One particular incident sticks in my mind. I had been inter-
viewing a doctor in a Manhattan hospital. I came out on the
street and hailed a cab. The cabby was a large man. No, let's
face it, he was dangerously overweight. We got talking.

"You a doctor?" he said.

"No, but I've been talking to doctors."

"Oh? What about?"

"Ill health. Obesity. Unfitness. And how to start improving
life by walking."

"My God," he said "I walk."

I was about to tell him about the book I was writing when
suddenly I noticed his picture in the permit on the dashboard.
It looked like a different man: slim and youthful. It must have
been taken years before. But no:

"It was only two years ago that that picture was taken."

"That's amazing. What's happened to make you put on so
much weight?"

"The magic of the moccasin still makes good medicine."
The New York Walk Book

So he told me his story. His name was Leonard Kommissar, and his parents came from Omsk, but he was Brooklyn born and bred. He had once been a heavy smoker. He had weighed less then, but was smoking himself into an early grave.

"I choked a fantastic amount. My God, I choked, and I coughed and coughed. I was smoking about three and a half packs a day – seventy or so a day. I also drank a lot of coffee. I tell you, I wound up doing myself more harm than I did any good there. I was on a highway one night and I had to pull over. I was choking for about four hours. Four hours! I really couldn't stop.

"Finally, I couldn't take it any more. There were three packs of cigarettes on the dashboard with my matches and a brand new lighter I had just bought. I rolled down the window and threw everything out. *Everything.* That was two years ago in June."

"And the weight?"

"I noticed that my craving after the first three or four weeks was to have something always in my mouth. A piece of chewing gum, a piece of cake, anything. Usually something sweet. I gained sixty-five pounds in two years."

Eventually he confronted his own obvious unfitness – he was only 45 – and finally sought medical advice. Now he was right at the start of a walking program.

Most people do not have such a straightforward problem. Their unfitness seldom amounts to the double, clear-cut extremities that confronted Leonard Kommissar within so short a time. They simply feel a need to be fitter than they are, and want to discover exactly what the problem is before seeking solutions.

It is possible now to measure fitness from a number of different points of view, to build an accurate fitness profile that can show you, as an individual, what you need to achieve or preserve basic fitness.

The first thing that I should say here is that fitness is notoriously difficult to measure. Whatever the accuracy of the figures mentioned later, there's one factor that defies scientific analysis: your feeling of personal well-being. As Ian Anderson says, "You can't measure well-ability."

Being slim and trim is supposed to give everyone an improved sense of well-being, but there are always the exceptions – those who refuse to feel ill or inferior simply because they do not conform to, say, the runner's ideal of physical fitness. I have a friend who stands 5′ 10″ and weighs a good 250 pounds. He has a zest for good food that is positively contagious. He drinks and smokes (though only in moderation). I have never known him to take any exercise at all. He runs his own business and has a psychological metabolism that seems continuously tuned to maximum. I get the impression that his emotional activity somehow spills over into his body, because he always seems to be glowing with health. His countenance is cherubic. "I thought I was overweight once," he remarked to me over a sumptuous lunch in a Thai restaurant. "I cut down my food and lost fifty pounds. I felt terrible. I didn't look good. So I gave it up." According to all the statistical tables, at 250 pounds he should not only feel sick, but he should feel discontented. Obstinately, he feels neither sick nor unhappy. A doctor would tell him that he's storing up trouble for himself later on. His reply would be that he would rather live happily for fifty-five years than ascetically for eighty. I haven't tried to persuade him to take up walking – and I don't think I will.

No, I can only talk to those who do feel a vague dissatisfaction about their way of life; those to whom the idea of extreme physical exertion is a threat, but who would, nevertheless, like to come to grips with their own obvious deficiencies.

But *do* you perceive your deficiencies? Dr. Roger Bannister, the first four-minute miler, has described fitness as "a state of mental and physical harmony, which enables someone to carry on his occupation to the best of his ability." But what constitutes "lack of harmony"? How do you quantify it?

Let us assume that you feel that not all is well with you. You don't exactly lead a puritan existence. You've never been one to aspire to being part of the physical elite, but you wouldn't mind doing a little something which may help you live to a ripe old age if you knew how much you had to do before you started and how long it was going to take to build a decent level of fitness. So, before I actually suggest ways of walking your way into a new level of health, let's see where you fit into the scale of things.

There is a small minority of people who should not consider any sort of an exercise program without consulting a doctor. Some authorities say that if you are sedentary and over 35, you should have a medical examination. Some even go so far as to say that everyone considering exercise, irrespective of age, should be medically screened. In an ideal world, perhaps; but in reality such a scheme would swamp the medical system. A mass of people needing exercise would take so long to get screened that they'd never actually begin. You can, however, screen yourself right now in a number of ways.

For instance, to establish a base line, you can assess your own risks of suffering a heart attack.

If you have your medical details at your fingertips, you can do your own assessment by turning to Appendix 1 of "The Walker's Yellow Pages," which represents the best estimates of fitness categories currently available. But if you're like me, you won't be able to remember what your blood pressure is, let alone what your cholesterol, triglycerides and glucose levels are, so why not start with the rough-and-ready-guide overleaf, which will help you answer the question: Am I at risk?

There is one more element of which you should be aware when assessing your own risk: stress. It has not been included in the table because it has so far proved impossible to assign numerical values to stress levels as against other factors, but most researchers now agree that stress does play a role in the onset of coronary disease. (It is also involved in the onset of disease and disability as a whole – including accidents – for reasons that are not yet completely understood.)

The relationship between stress and heart disease has been established in only one set of conditions – driving – the result of work done at London's Middlesex Hospital by Dr. Peter Taggart

---

"There is a leisure about walking, no matter what pace you set, that lets down the tension."

Hal Borland, *To Own the Streets and Fields*

ARE YOU AT RISK?

The following table, adapted from one devised by the Michigan Heart Association, is a rough guide to help you determine whether or not your current life style is increasing the chances of your having a heart attack. Simply record the figure that applies to you in each category, tally up your score and assess your risk by seeing where you fit into this scale:

  5–9 : well below average risk   26–32: high risk
  10–14: below average risk   33–47: extremely high risk
  15–25: average risk

WARNING: If you are a smoker who inhales deeply and you smoke your cigarette down to a short butt, add one to your total. When assessing the hereditary factor, count only parents, grand-parents, brothers and sisters and relatives. If you are at "high risk," see a doctor before you undertake any exercise program, and try to see one anyway within the next few weeks. If you fall in the "extremely high risk" category, don't take any chances: if you haven't recently done so, see a doctor immediately.

SEX	Female under 40 1	Female 40–50 2	Female over 50 3	Male 5	Stocky male 6	Bald, stocky male 7
EXERCISE	Intensive work and recreational exertion 2	Moderately active work and recreational exertion 2	Sedentary work and extended or intense recreational exertion 3	Sedentary work and moderate recreational exertion 5	Sedentary work and light recreational exertion 6	Complete lack of all exercise 8
TOBACCO SMOKING	Non-user 0	Cigar and/ or pipe 1	10 cigarettes or less a day 2	20 cigarettes a day 4	30 cigarettes a day 6	40 a day or more 10
WEIGHT	More than 5lb. below standard weight 0	−5 to +5lb. standard weight 1	6–20lb. overweight 2	21–35lb. overweight 3	36–50lb. overweight 5	51–65lb. overweight 7
HEREDITY	No known history of heart disease 1	1 relative over 60 with cardio-vascular disease 2	2 relatives over 60 with cardio-vascular disease 3	1 relative under 60 with cardio-vascular disease 4	2 relatives under 60 with cardio-vascular disease 6	3 relatives under 60 with cardio-vascular disease 7
AGE	10 to 20 1	21 to 30 2	31 to 40 3	41 to 50 4	51 to 60 5	61 and over 8

"No cold nor chill, nor ache nor pain, can survive a few hours walking, and all one's cares and worries go the same way."
A. N. Cooper, *A Holiday on Tramp*

and his team. They found that stress releases large quantities of the hormone noradrenalin into the bloodstream. This reaction is accompanied by raised levels of fatty acids, which are associated with the formation of atheroma, the sludgy substance that clogs arteries and eventually leads to atherosclerosis and thrombosis.

Statistically, the most dramatic association between stress and a heart attack occurs after bereavement. In the first six months after the death of a spouse, the death rate among the surviving partners is higher than would otherwise be expected – up to 40 percent for widowers. Nearly 5 percent of widowers aged over 45 die within six months of the death of their wife, mainly from heart disease – victims, almost literally, of broken hearts.

It was this fact that gave a US naval psychiatrist, Lieutenant Commander Richard Rahe, a base line against which he could compare the stress imposed by a number of other "life situations." He devised a number of questions for his patients, and from their answers he calculated a stress index. He found that the average stress index was about 30 and that coronary patients tended to have an increase in their stress indices in the two years before their attack, and that the severity of the attack was proportional to the final level of their indices. It is interesting – and important – to note that he took into account the idea that stress is not always related to traditionally negative events. Promotion, an increase in salary, vacations, Christmas: these are all welcome, but all stressful events.

The Rahe Stress Index is worth reproducing (p. 65) because it will give you a rough idea of any recent or long-term strains that you may be operating under. It *is*, however, very rough. When I first did it, I was harsh on myself, and my score showed me that I was living under a permanent strain equivalent to the death of several spouses. Hastily, I repeated the test, and found that I was not overstressed after all. In addition, the degree to which one is affected by any of the conditions varies with individuals. It is well established, for instance, that so-called Type A individuals – people who are ambitious, aggressive, impatient and go-ahead – are more at risk than the easy-going Type Bs, who don't get uptight at work or worry about their mortgages. Still, the test is worth doing: it is of interest in itself; and, in addition, if it shows you that you *are* highly stressed, then it is an indication that you should consider building some activity into your life – like an extended walking program – which will help you to relieve your stress, both mentally and physically, no matter how otherwise fit you think you are.

If you decide that you had better have a medical checkup, ensure that your doctor has the equipment to give you a stress test. There's no denying it cuts a lot of corners. After one consultation, you will have gained all the information necessary to provide you with an accurate fitness profile and a safe exercise prescription – information that it might take you several hours of careful work to obtain at home.

Stress testing is now an established part of medical procedure and many millions of people have undergone it. For those of you who have not, the name may sound somewhat off-putting. As Dr. Sam Fox, one of America's leading cardiologists, put it to me in his consulting room in Georgetown Hospital in Washington, D.C.: "Stress is considered bad news in many of its connotations. And tests are things we never like to see in school or university. In the mind of a lay person, 'stress testing' may conjure up unhappy thoughts. I prefer to call the test a 'tolerance evaluation.'"

Whatever you prefer to call it, the routine is perfectly simple. The doctor will take down your medical history, give you a physical examination where he or she will take your blood pressure, check your smoking and drinking habits, assess your cholesterol level, measure the amount of fat you have as compared to muscle, and of course take an electrocardiogram (ECG or EKG – both abbreviations are in use). This is an electrical tracing of the heart's activities, during which you will be subjected to increasing levels of strain.

The stressing – sorry, "tolerance evaluation" – is done on a treadmill, which should, in a few years, be one of the most familiar objects in a doctor's consulting room. It consists of a rubber belt wound around rollers at each end of a flat surface, wired to a speedometer and to a brake which can be used to

THE RAHE STRESS INDEX

Have any of these events happened to you over the last six months? Tally up your score for each event that applies and check your total with the scoring guide below to see if your life is dangerously overstressful.

1. Death of spouse	**100**	
2. Divorce	**73**	
3. Marital separation	**65**	
4. Jail term	**63**	
5. Death of close family member	**63**	
6. Personal injury or illness	**53**	
7. Marriage	**50**	
8. Fired at work	**47**	
9. Marital reconciliation	**45**	
10. Retirement	**45**	
11. Change in health of family member	**44**	
12. Pregnancy	**40**	
13. Sex difficulties	**39**	
14. Gain of new family member	**39**	
15. Business readjustment	**39**	
16. Change in financial state	**38**	
17. Death of close friend	**37**	
18. Change to different line of work	**36**	
19. Change in number of arguments with spouse	**35**	
20. A large mortgage or loan	**31**	
21. Foreclosure of mortgage or loan	**30**	
22. Change in responsibilities at work	**29**	
23. Son or daughter leaving home	**29**	
24. Trouble with in-laws	**29**	
25. Outstanding personal achievement	**28**	
26. Spouse begins or stops work	**26**	
27. Begin or end school or college	**26**	
28. Change in living conditions	**25**	
29. A change in personal habits	**24**	
30. Trouble with the boss	**23**	
31. Change in work hours or conditions	**20**	
32. Change in residence	**20**	
33. Change in school or college	**20**	
34. Change in recreation	**19**	
35. Change in church activities	**19**	
36. Change in social activities	**18**	
37. A moderate mortgage or loan	**17**	
38. Change in sleeping habits	**16**	
39. Change in number of family get-togethers	**15**	
40. Change in eating habits	**15**	
41. Holiday	**13**	
42. Christmas	**12**	
43. Minor violations of the law	**11**	

Below 60: Your life has been unusually free from stress lately.

60 to 80: You have had a normal amount of stress recently. This score is average for the ordinary wear and tear of life.

80 to 100: The stress in your life is a little high, probably because of one recent event.

100 upwards: Pressures are piling up, either at home or work, or both. You are under serious stress, and the higher you score above 100 the worse the strain.

increase resistance and thus simulate an increasing gradient. Going through all its paces, the treadmill can put you through the slowest of slow walks to a sprint up a mountain.

Before you step on the treadmill, you will be wired up to the ECG. It takes about ten minutes to work up to your limit – your "maximal" heartbeat – and at the end of that time, you will probably be sweating and panting as if you've been forcing yourself up a mountainside, around a track, or back and forth across a squash court.

This may sound a forbidding, even dangerous exercise for those with a potential heart condition, but it isn't. For one thing if you're getting on in years or you're very unfit, you won't be able to do that much. Whatever your state, the doctors can use the pinpoint accuracy of the ECG to stop you short of exhaustion or danger. The possibility of someone having a fatal heart attack as a result of undergoing a stress test is extremely remote. The US Air Force has, in the course of several years, arranged for the testing of over fifteen thousand physically untrained men between 17 and 62. During the course of the testing, they experienced only one heart attack, suffered by a

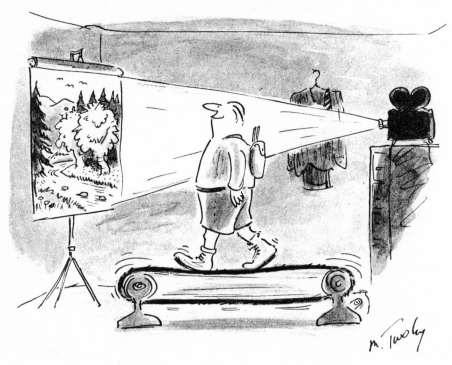

51-year-old man, and that occurred not during the test but thirty minutes after it.

It is true that of the tens of thousands of people who undergo stress testing each year, a good number of them may well be at risk; in short, there is bound to be the occasional crisis. Statistics show that one in ten thousand will develop some sort of heart trouble during the test. But the trouble might have developed anyway; and where better to have an attack, if you're going to have one, than in a doctor's office?

Ian Anderson had the unnerving experience of seeing an unfit patient go into total collapse. "It was extremely frightening," he told me, "he just keeled over without any warning. His heart stopped. The ECG was just showing a straight line. For a few seconds he was as good as dead. If he hadn't been walking on the treadmill, wired up to the ECG, he would have been. As it was, we applied immediate resuscitation. He recovered, and has now begun to exercise again."

Just How Fit Are You?

Assuming you are not in dire need of a full checkup, it is perfectly possible to get an idea of your own fitness level. It may take a little longer to discover some basic truths about yourself, but it is more fun. From there, you can set up your own walking program, get your fitness up to a satisfactory level, and indeed go on safely from there into any number of more demanding activities.

As in a doctor's consulting room, your pulse will take you right to the heart of the matter. In Appendix 2 of "The Walker's Yellow Pages" you will find tables that rank a cross section of the population by sex, age and a number of standard fitness measurements. You can use these statistics to find out how the measurements you are about to take on yourself compare with those of the rest of the population.

Stage 1: Determining Your Resting Heartbeat
The first thing you need to do is take your resting heartbeat, or pulse. There are a number of places you can use to take your own pulse: the artery just inside your wrist bone; the carotid artery on the side of the throat, either just above the collarbone or just below the jaw (don't press too hard, though, and never

press on both sides at once, otherwise you cut down the blood supply to the brain); the artery that runs through the temple; or over the heart itself.

Probably the easiest is at the wrist. Place two fingers on your wrist and look at your watch. The pulse is usually measured in terms of beats per minute, but you don't have to count for a whole minute. Count for fifteen seconds and multiply by four. (Theoretically you can do it for any amount of time as long as you can multiply the result to make a beats-per-minute count, but if you do it for much less than fifteen seconds you will find you have to begin estimating half beats or quarter beats to get an accurate figure.)

To record your resting heartbeat, sit quietly for several minutes, breathing gently. As you will see from the tables in Appendix 2 of "The Walker's Yellow Pages," resting heart-beats for people of "average" fitness (30th–60th percentiles) vary widely: from 72 for women in their 40s, down to 58 for men in their 40s. The thing to remember is that the lower your resting heartbeat, the fitter you are (unless it's the result of disease). Some highly trained endurance runners have hearts that beat less than forty times a minute. If your resting pulse is much over 90, though, you probably haven't got a great deal of spare capacity. Try to see your doctor soon.

From the tables you can also see what your theoretical maximum heart rate is. By taking 85 percent of this figure, you can, in addition, work out what your *practical* maximum should be, assuming you wish to drive yourself that hard.

Stage 2: Determining Your Fitness

To do this you have to stretch yourself a little, at the same time keeping a close watch on your own pulse. The best method to use is a step test. A number of tests have been devised which advocate different combinations of step height (according to your own height and/or weight) and speed. Some of these tests have a major defect: you have to be extremely fit in order to do them at all. One such test is the famous Harvard Step Test, included in James Fixx's *Complete Book of Running*. It tells me, as a six-footer, to choose a step twenty inches high, and to step up and down it once every two seconds for four minutes. Twenty inches is *very* high, I discovered. My heart could take it, but my legs couldn't. I collapsed with aching thighs after $2\frac{1}{2}$

minutes. Rather than put you through this kind of agony, I'll steer you to two other tests, one by which you can assess your fitness at a very basic level, and another more demanding one, with more carefully quantified results.

Step Test 1: For Basic Fitness The most practical test to establish for yourself your basic level of fitness appears in Laurence Morehouse and Leonard Gross's *Total Fitness in 30 Minutes a Week.* Its advantages are two-fold: it involves body weight (rather than height); and it allows steps that range between seven and twelve inches high. This means that you can take the test equally well with a pile of books, a stool, a chair, a flight of steps, a bench or whatever else is at your disposal. Look at the table below, find your approximate weight and then match it to the column beneath the height of the step you are thinking of using. This will give you the number of steps you should be taking per minute.

STEP TEST 1							
Stepping Rate (steps per minute)							
		Height of Step (inches)					
		7	8	9	10	11	12
Body Weight (Pounds)	100	30	30	30	30	30	30
	120	30	30	30	30	30	30
	140	30	30	30	30	20	20
	160	30	30	30	20	20	20
	180	30	30	20	20	20	20
	200	30	20	20	20	20	20
	220	20	20	20	20	20	20

I weigh 173 pounds, and at the moment of writing I have at hand the two-volume *Shorter Oxford English Dictionary* and *Gray's Anatomy,* suitably uplifting bodies of knowledge which also happen to measure just seven inches high when stacked up on the floor. If I were to repeat the test, I'd be stepping at the rate of 30 per minute.

Having selected your step and your rhythm, simply step on and off it for one minute. You can change your lead leg from time to time if you want to. Keep a check on your pace in the first ten seconds. Each step will take either two or three seconds and you should find it easy to get into a rhythm.

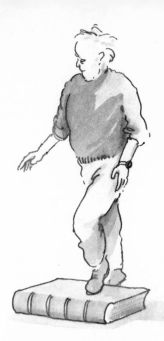

As you start, listen to what your body is telling you. If there is any indication that all is not well – heavy sweating, muscle cramps, heart palpitations, difficulty in breathing – stop!

After a minute of stepping, stop, sit down, and take your pulse for fifteen seconds. However fit you are, the test will have raised your pulse to some extent and you may find it easier to count it by placing your hand on your heart, rather than feeling for it at your wrist. If it's 120 or over – that is, 30 or over in a fifteen-second period – your tolerance is low. Stop right there.

If it's under 120, repeat the exercise, allowing no more than half a minute's rest. Repeat the sequence three times in all, then rest for a minute and take your pulse one last time.

If your pulse did not reach 30 per fifteen-second period (120 per minute) in the course of the exercises, and if in the one minute's rest at the end it declined by at least ten beats per minute (i.e., if your final fifteen-second count was no more than 20), you're fundamentally sound and fit enough to undertake the basic walking program discussed in the next chapter.

"Afoot and light-hearted I take to the open road,
Healthy, free, the world before me,
The long brown path before me leading wherever I choose."
Walt Whitman, "The Song of the Open Road"

Step Test 2: For a More Detailed Assessment If you want to get a more precise fix on your level of fitness, try this step test advocated by Michael Pollack, Jack Wilmore and Sam Fox in their book *Health and Fitness through Physical Activity*. Find a bench or a chair about sixteen inches high and step on and off it for a total of three minutes. Men should step at the rate of twenty-four steps per minute (six steps every fifteen seconds) and women at the rate of twenty-two steps per minute. At the end of three minutes, take your pulse rate and compare it with the following table:

RESPONSE TO STEP TEST 2

Percentile Rankings	Heart Rate: Women	Men	Percentile Rankings	Heart Rate: Women	Men
99	128	120	50	166	156
90	148	128	40	170	162
80	156	140	30	172	166
70	160	148	20	180	172
60	163	152	10	184	178

A word of warning: This is quite a tough exercise. At the lower end of the scale, the heart rates actually exceed the maximum recommended rates shown in Appendix 2 of "The Walker's Yellow Pages." If your maximum heart rate can exceed 178 for a man or 184 for a woman, fine. If not don't try this second step test until you've hardened up a bit.

Other Paces You Can Put Yourself Through
Of course there are a number of other ways of assessing your fitness, in addition to measuring your pulse rate. If you share the common urge to compare your performance to that of others, you may like to try the next two tests.

The Push-up Men should perform this exercise holding their bodies as rigidly as possible, angling up from the toes and bending the arms until the chest just touches the ground. Women should use a modified position, pushing up from their knees. You can compare your performance with the table of standards overleaf. (The categories are very approximate, as nobody has yet seen fit to gather statistics representative of the population as a whole.)

PUSH-UPS (no time limit): MALES					
AGE	EXCELLENT	GOOD	AVERAGE	FAIR	POOR
20–29	55 & over	45–54	35–44	20–34	0–19
30–39	45 & over	35–44	25–34	15–24	0–14
40–49	40 & over	30–39	20–29	12–19	0–11
50–59	35 & over	25–34	15–24	8–14	0–7
60–69	30 & over	20–29	10–19	5–9	0–4

PUSH-UPS (no time limit): FEMALES (Modified push-up)					
AGE	EXCELLENT	GOOD	AVERAGE	FAIR	POOR
20–29	49 & over	34–48	17–33	6–16	0–5
30–39	40 & over	25–39	12–24	4–11	0–3
40–49	35 & over	20–34	8–19	3–7	0–2
50–59	30 & over	15–29	6–14	2–5	0–1
60–69	20 & over	5–19	3–4	1–2	0

Sit-ups (Stomach Curls) Put your hands behind your head, tuck your feet under a piece of solid furniture (or get somebody to hold your feet), crook your knees a little and then see how many times in a minute you can curl up from the floor and touch your elbows to your thighs. Again, you can compare your performance to the approximate table of standards.

SIT-UPS (per minute): MALES					
AGE	EXCELLENT	GOOD	AVERAGE	FAIR	POOR
20–29	48 & over	43–47	37–42	33–36	0–32
30–39	40 & over	35–39	29–34	25–28	0–24
40–49	35 & over	30–34	24–29	20–23	0–19
50–59	30 & over	25–29	19–24	15–18	0–14
60–69	25 & over	20–24	14–19	10–13	0–9

SIT-UPS (per minute): FEMALES					
AGE	EXCELLENT	GOOD	AVERAGE	FAIR	POOR
20–29	44 & over	39–43	33–38	29–32	0–28
30–39	36 & over	31–35	25–30	21–24	0–20
40–49	31 & over	26–30	19–25	16–18	0–15
50–59	26 & over	21–25	15–20	11–14	0–10
60–69	21 & over	16–20	10–15	6–9	0–5

Fit or Fat?

Finally, I'd like to help you to answer a question that almost everyone asks themselves at some time or another and which for countless thousands of people (and scores of magazines and newspapers) is positively obsessive: Am I too fat?

Put in this form, the question is so vague that it is both unhelpful and unnerving. Being a *little* fat is not a problem – everyone has a certain percentage of fat on their bodies. Some people, though, are disastrously obese. It would be nice to know where you fit on this scale before you decide whether you want to do anything about it or not. So let's rephrase the question to read: *How* fat am I?

It is a question worth worrying about. Surveys in London general practices have shown that, overall, 56 percent of the women and 52 percent of the men were at least 15 percent above their ideal weight. The risks of carrying about too much fat are considerable. The fatter you are, the more likely it is that you will die earlier than would be expected, as the table below demonstrates.

THE RISKS OF BEING OVERWEIGHT						
	Men			Women		
Percent overweight	10%	20%	30%	10%	20%	30%
Increased chance of shorter life expectancy	20%	30%	40%	9%	20%	30%

As we saw in the previous chapter, fat people are more prone to diseases of the heart and blood vessels. They are also more prone to diabetes, to strained joints and ligaments, and to arthritis and back pain.

The cause of obesity is quite simple. Our bodies derive energy from the food and drink that we consume. The creation of fat is the body's response to a surplus of energy, which plainly and simply means that we get fat by eating too much. This is true even in those extremely rare cases where gland troubles – endocrine disorders – are present. Certainly, such disorders can accentuate a tendency toward obesity, but it still remains true that the sufferer has eaten more than he or she needs. There is still the same imbalance between intake and output. Nobody has yet managed to starve themselves into obesity. As a nutritionist friend of mine once said, rather brutally, when I asked him why I was beginning to put on weight: "Fat comes from food. There's nowhere else it *can* come from."

Typically the gain occurs insidiously. Only one hundred calories above your requirements every day – the equivalent of two slices of bread or a medium-size boiled potato – can result in a weight gain of ten pounds a year. If continued, such a minute excess would result in a staggering fifty-pound burden of fat at the end of five years.

To those who tend to put on fat easily, this explanation, though true, is far too simple to be emotionally acceptable all at once. "Why do you let yourself put on weight?" seems as unfair a question as one put to me by my bank manager when I was a student (and repeated at significant periods by other bank managers over the years): "How is it, Mr. Man, that you consistently spend more than you earn?" To answer the question and then to act upon it demands a totally new outlook on life, for the root cause involves habits so regular and so ingrained that they are largely unconscious. The sufferers know they should change, yet how *can* they as long as they live in a society that expects them to eat three meals a day and offers countless opportunities to snack on all sorts of calorie-laden junk foods and to consume substantial amounts of alcohol at the slightest hint of an appropriate business or social occasion?

The first step in coping with the problem is to analyze it. Standard weight tables like the ones shown here are a good starting point. They were devised by the Metropolitan Life Insurance Company, and they give a rough guide to average weights of a representative cross section of the population. But they are no more than a starting point. Firstly, they are very rough. You have to decide whether you have a small, medium or large frame. Secondly, each category has a range of up to twenty-two pounds. This is fine for insurance actuaries, but in personal terms it's pretty wide. According to the tables, two medium-framed women of the same height can differ by thirteen pounds. But what the tables do *not* show is that one may have a much higher percentage of fat on her body and thus experience continual worries about how she looks, how fit she is and how fit she ought to be. Men such as college football players or stocky middle-aged men are often overweight in terms of the tables, but they are not necessarily unfit.

DESIRABLE WEIGHTS (IN POUNDS)				
Group	Height (with shoes on)	Small Frame	Medium Frame	Large Frame
Men (1-inch heels)	5' 2"	112–120	118–129	126–141
	5' 3"	115–123	121–133	129–144
	5' 4"	118–126	124–136	132–148
	5' 5"	121–129	127–139	135–152
	5' 6"	124–133	130–143	138–156
	5' 7"	128–137	134–147	142–161
	5' 8"	132–141	138–152	147–166
	5' 9"	136–145	142–156	151–170
	5' 10"	140–150	146–160	155–174
	5' 11"	144–154	150–165	159–179
	6' 0"	148–158	154–170	164–184
	6' 1"	152–162	158–175	168–189
	6' 2"	156–167	162–180	173–194
	6' 3"	160–171	167–185	178–199
	6' 4"	164–175	172–190	182–204
Women* (2-inch heels)	4' 10"	92– 98	96–107	104–119
	4' 11"	94–101	98–110	106–122
	5' 0"	96–104	101–113	109–125
	5' 1"	99–107	104–116	112–128
	5' 2"	102–110	107–119	115–131
	5' 3"	105–113	110–112	118–134
	5' 4"	108–116	113–116	121–138
	5' 5"	111–119	116–130	125–142
	5' 6"	114–123	120–135	129–146
	5' 7"	118–127	124–139	133–150
	5' 8"	122–131	128–143	137–154
	5' 9"	126–135	132–147	141–158
	5' 10"	130–140	136–151	145–163
	5' 11"	134–144	140–155	149–168
	6' 0"	138–148	144–159	153–173

*For women between 18 and 25, subtract one pound for each year under 25.
Source: Metropolitan Life Insurance Company, 1959.

The real point at issue is not whether you are overweight or not but whether you are *overfat*. Fat weight can be expressed as a percentage of the individual's total body weight. Typically, nonsporting males between 18 and 28 weigh about 165 pounds, of which 16 percent is fat. Nonsporting males in their 40s weigh around 180 pounds, of which 23 percent is fat. As a person ages, the increase in his or her weight is almost always due to an increase in fat – fat that a middle-aged man or woman could well do without.

The widely accepted proportions of fat to body weight – or "The Fat Continuum," as I like to think of it – are as follows:

	Men	Women
Ideal Level	16–19%	22–25%
Danger Level	25% and above	35% and above

Assessing Your Fat Content

There are a number of popularly recommended methods for determining whether you are too fat or not. You can stand in front of a mirror and judge for yourself, honestly, whether you approve of the way your flesh hangs. Try jiggling up and down a bit; if you go out of focus, you have a problem.

Or you can do the "inch-of-pinch" test. Find a book an inch thick, then take the flesh at the side of your waist or at the back of your upper arm between your thumb and index finger. Keeping your thumb as rigid as possible, take your hand away and compare the distance between thumb and finger with the book. If either fold is more than an inch thick, you're probably overfat. Each inch is estimated to equal forty pounds of fat, but that in itself doesn't tell you much until you have worked it out as a percentage of your total body weight. Anyway, like the mirror test, it can really only tell you if you have a problem, not what *type* of a problem you have.

Assessing the fat content of your own body accurately is not easy. If you really want to go all out, you have to get yourself weighed underwater – a procedure normally used only for research purposes. The theory of underwater weighing is based on the fact that bone and muscle sink, while fat floats. Of two people who weigh the same on land, the fatter of the two weighs less in water. But since in order to be weighed underwater you need a specially built vat or swimming pool with overhead apparatus, the system is hardly the practical answer for home use.

For Men Only

For men, it is relatively simple to calculate the percentage of body fat. There are two methods.

Method 1: The first and simplest of the two is based on the fact that the amount of fat around a man's waist fairly represents the amount of fat on his body as a whole. Using the table below, match your body weight to your waist girth with a ruler and read off your fat percentage on the scale in the center of the chart. A 170-pound man, with a 34-inch waist, has a body that is 18 percent fat (this is the example shown by the dotted line on the diagram). A 205-pounder with a 40-inch waist is 25 percent fat. With a 33.5-inch waist, tipping the scales at 173 pounds, I test out at 16.5 percent fat.

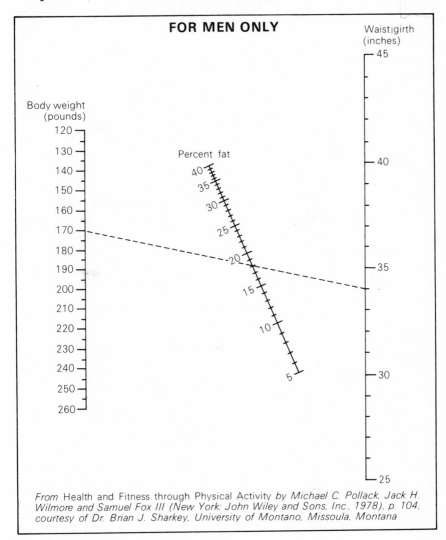

FOR MEN ONLY

Waist girth (inches)

Body weight (pounds)

Percent fat

From Health and Fitness through Physical Activity by Michael C. Pollack, Jack H. Wilmore and Samuel Fox III (New York: John Wiley and Sons, Inc., 1978), p. 104, courtesy of Dr. Brian J. Sharkey, University of Montana, Missoula, Montana

Method 2: The second method involves a little mathematics. It was devised by B. C. Frederick, editor of the US magazine *Running*, who says that it is accurate to within 2 percent for all but the lankiest or fattest of men. It is based on what he calls a Ponderal Index, which is a ratio of height to weight. The ratio is calculated by dividing your height in inches by the cube root of your weight in pounds:

$$\text{Ponderal Index} = \text{Height (in inches)} \div \sqrt[3]{\text{Weight (in pounds)}}$$

For convenience, here are some approximate cube roots (for greater accuracy use a calculator):

118 lbs. = 4.9	141 lbs. = 5.2	166 lbs. = 5.5	195 lbs. = 5.8
125 lbs. = 5.0	149 lbs. = 5.3	175 lbs. = 5.6	205 lbs. = 5.9
133 lbs. = 5.1	157 lbs. = 5.4	185 lbs. = 5.7	216 lbs. = 6.0

Once you have worked out your Ponderal Index, read it off against the scale below to find out your percentage of body fat. For example, at the time of writing, I weigh 173 pounds and I am six feet tall (72 inches). The cube root of 173 is 5.575. $72 \div 5.575 = 12.91$, giving me a fat ratio of 15.5 percent, which as it happens, correlates pretty well with the result of the first test.

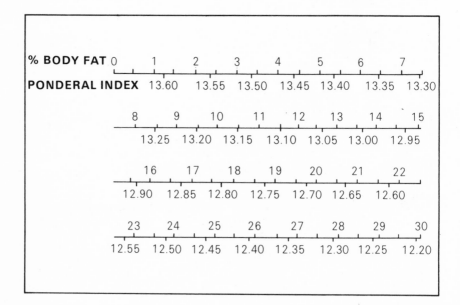

For Women Only

Assessing a woman's body composition is much more tricky. Women have a much greater variety of shape than men because their fat distribution is less regular. Sometimes the weight sinks to the bottom; sometimes it builds up on thighs or arms or breasts. Some women are trim above the waist and large below it. To balance out the variety of factors involved you will actually need to measure skin folds at and below your waist with the help of a pair of skin-fold calipers, small pincers calibrated to measure the distance between the pincers in millimeters.

A Note on Calipers: Skin-fold calipers are theoretically very simple devices. They should have two pincers, or arms, that lock onto the fold of skin in such a way that you can record the gap in between the two pincers. Ideally, they should have a millimeter scale attached. Unfortunately, there is no great public demand for calipers specifically designed for the purpose we have in mind. Ask for skin-fold calipers and you will probably be presented with a luxury object designed to exact the maximum possible price from the medical profession. In England, for instance, a typical pair costs no less than £78 (close to $150). I have in my possession a pair that cost me

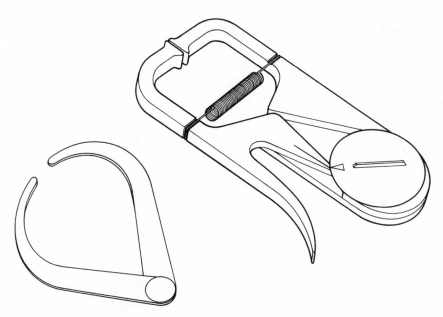

50 pence ($1), but they are no longer on the market. You can, however, buy ordinary, inexpensive calipers such as the kind used by carpenters or engineers. If they do not have a scale attached, all you do is take the measurement (firmly enough so that the arms hold the flesh without pinching) and then, with the help of a metric ruler, calculate the distance between the tips of the pincers. The tips may not be comfortably padded, but the device will do the job well enough.

How to Proceed
Step 1: Women below 40 should measure the skin folds at the front of the lower thigh (a little above the knee) and at the waist (on your side just above the hip bone). Women 40 and above should measure the folds at the side of the chest just beneath the armpit and at the front of the thigh just above the knee.

Step 2: When you have noted the two measurements, consult the table appropriate to your age category on p. 81, find the correct figure for each skin fold and note the conversion factor next to it.

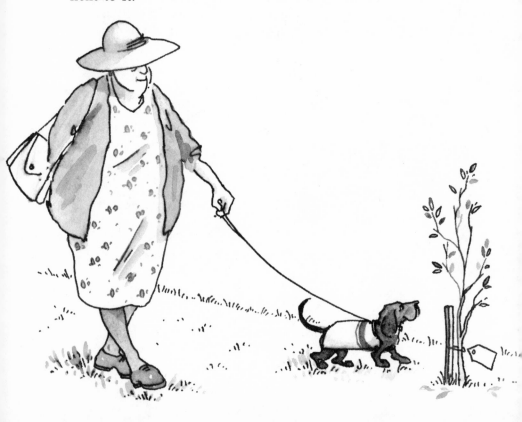

SKIN-FOLD CONVERSION FACTORS Women under 40

	WAIST FOLD				THIGH FOLD		
Fold (mm)	Conversion	Fold (mm)	Conversion	Fold (mm)	Conversion	Fold (mm)	Conversion
6	1.0804	26	1.0644	6	0.0066	26	0.0286
7	1.0796	27	1.0636	7	0.0077	27	0.0297
8	1.0788	28	1.0628	8	0.0088	28	0.0308
9	1.0780	29	1.0620	9	0.0099	29	0.0319
10	1.0772	30	1.0612	10	0.0110	30	0.0330
11	1.0764	31	1.0604	11	0.0121	31	0.0331
12	1.0756	32	1.0596	12	0.0132	32	0.0352
13	1.0748	33	1.0588	13	0.0143	33	0.0363
14	1.0740	34	1.0580	14	0.0154	34	0.0374
15	1.0732	35	1.0572	15	0.0165	35	0.0385
16	1.0724	36	1.0564	16	0.0176	36	0.0396
17	1.0716	37	1.0556	17	0.0187	37	0.0407
18	1.0708	38	1.0548	18	0.0198	38	0.0418
19	1.0700	39	1.0540	19	0.0209	39	0.0429
20	1.0692	40	1.0532	20	0.0220	40	0.0440
21	1.0684	41	1.0524	21	0.0231	41	0.0451
22	1.0676	42	1.0516	22	0.0242	42	0.0462
23	1.0668	43	1.0508	23	0.0253	43	0.0473
24	1.0660	44	1.0500	24	0.0264	44	0.0484
25	1.0652	45	1.0492	25	0.0275	45	0.0495

SKIN-FOLD CONVERSION FACTORS Women 40 and Above

	CHEST FOLD				THIGH FOLD		
Fold (mm)	Conversion	Fold (mm)	Conversion	Fold (mm)	Conversion	Fold (mm)	Conversion
6	1.0682	26	1.0442	6	0.0042	26	0.0182
7	1.0670	27	1.0430	7	0.0049	27	0.0189
8	1.0658	28	1.0418	8	0.0056	28	0.0196
9	1.0646	29	1.0406	9	0.0063	29	0.0203
10	1.0634	30	1.0394	10	0.0070	30	0.0210
11	1.0622	31	1.0382	11	0.0077	31	0.0217
12	1.0610	32	1.0370	12	0.0084	32	0.0224
13	1.0598	33	1.0358	13	0.0091	33	0.0231
14	1.0586	34	1.0346	14	0.0098	34	0.0238
15	1.0574	35	1.0334	15	0.0105	35	0.0245
16	1.0562	36	1.0322	16	0.0112	36	0.0252
17	1.0550	37	1.0310	17	0.0119	37	0.0259
18	1.0538	38	1.0298	18	0.0126	38	0.0266
19	1.0526	39	1.0286	19	0.0133	39	0.0273
20	1.0514	40	1.0274	20	0.0140	40	0.0280
21	1.0502	41	1.0262	21	0.0147	41	0.0287
22	1.0490	42	1.0250	22	0.0154	42	0.0294
23	1.0478	43	1.0238	23	0.0161	43	0.0301
24	1.0466	44	1.0226	24	0.0168	44	0.0308
25	1.0454	45	1.0214	25	0.0175	45	0.0315

WALK!

BODY DENSITY CONVERSION TABLE

DENSITY	PERCENT FAT	DENSITY	PERCENT FAT
1.010	40.10	1.049	21.88
1.011	39.61	1.050	21.43
1.012	39.13	1.051	20.98
1.013	38.65	1.052	20.53
1.014	38.17	1.053	20.09
1.015	37.68	1.054	19.64
1.016	37.20	1.055	19.19
1.017	36.73	1.056	18.75
1.018	36.25	1.057	18.31
1.019	35.77	1.058	17.86
1.020	35.29	1.059	17.42
1.021	34.82	1.060	16.98
1.022	34.34	1.061	16.54
1.023	33.87	1.062	16.10
1.024	33.40	1.063	15.66
1.025	32.93	1.064	15.23
1.026	32.46	1.065	14.79
1.027	31.99	1.066	14.35
1.028	31.52	1.067	13.92
1.029	31.05	1.068	13.48
1.030	30.58	1.069	13.05
1.031	30.12	1.070	12.62
1.032	29.65	1.071	12.18
1.033	29.19	1.072	11.75
1.034	28.72	1.073	11.32
1.035	28.26	1.074	10.89
1.036	27.80	1.075	10.47
1.037	27.34	1.076	10.04
1.038	26.88	1.077	9.61
1.039	26.42	1.078	9.18
1.040	25.96	1.079	8.76
1.041	25.50	1.080	8.33
1.042	25.05	1.081	7.91
1.043	24.59	1.082	7.49
1.044	24.14	1.083	7.06
1.045	23.68	1.084	6.64
1.046	23.23	1.085	6.22
1.047	22.78	1.086	5.80
1.048	22.33	1.087	5.38

Tables developed by M. L. Pollack (Institute for Aerobics Research) and A. J. Jackson (University of Houston). Reproduced, with permission, from Health and Fitness through Physical Activity by Michael L. Pollack, Jack H. Wilmore and Samuel Fox III (New York: John Wiley and Sons, 1978).

Step 3: Women under 40 should then subtract their thigh conversion factor from their waist conversion factor. Women 40 and above should subtract their thigh conversion factor from their chest conversion factor. The result will be your body density (in grams per cubic centimeter).

Step 4: Finally, check the Body Density Table opposite and read off your fat percentage.

For instance, if you are a young woman with waist and thigh skin folds of 24mm and 20mm respectively, you'll see from the first table on p. 81 that the conversion figures are 1.0660 and 0.0220. Take the second figure from the first, giving you a density of 1.0440, which, if you look at the Body Density Table opposite is the equivalent to 24.14 percent fat. If you think this all sounds complicated . . . you're right! But it does work.

By now, if you're still with me, you should have gained a pretty clear idea of how sound you are in heart, limb and flesh. If you're unhappy with the result, read on for a program that *could* change your life. If you're happy with the way you are, read on anyway and I'll show you how to stay that way.

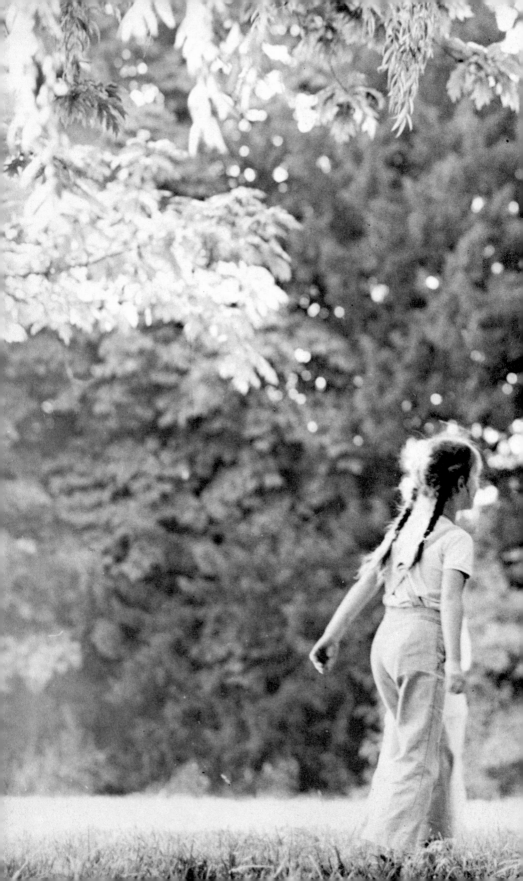

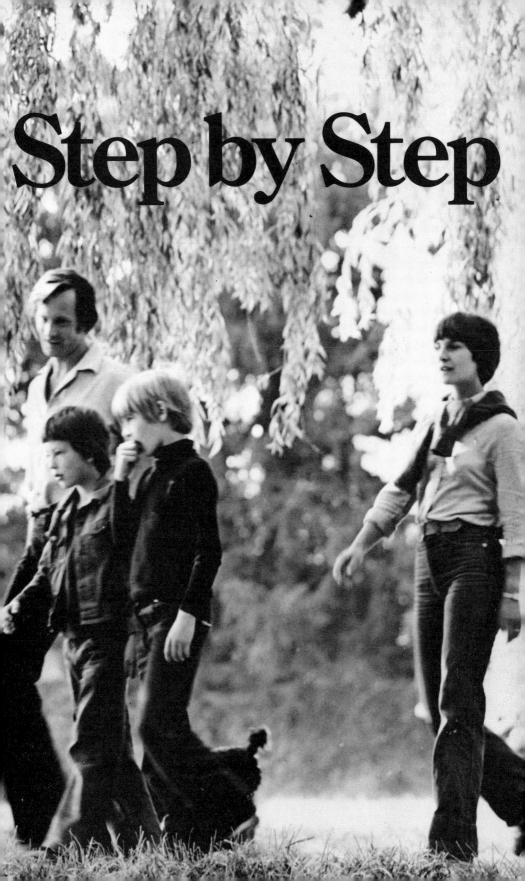

Step by Step

Step by Step

IN "THE WALKER'S YELLOW PAGES" at the end of the book, you'll find a series of suggested walking programs that will build you a basic level of fitness. This chapter is an introduction to it. Since the program is mainly intended for those who are unused to exercise, maybe a little overweight, perhaps middle-aged plus, it's worthwhile underlining the two principles upon which the program is based:

1. Take it easy,
   and
2. Build up at a slow, steady pace.

The dangers of starting too eagerly were effectively, if unintentionally, underlined as a result of a campaign initiated by John F. Kennedy. He happened on a 1908 Executive Order of Theodore Roosevelt, another physical fitness fanatic, suggesting that the Marines ought to be able to hike fifty miles in under three days. In February 1963, concerned that the new generation to which "the torch had been passed" (to quote him in a quite different context) might not be able to carry it very far, Kennedy challenged the Marines – and anyone else – to undertake the task.

The Kennedy enthusiasm proved as infectious as he had hoped. A number of Marines rose to the occasion and successfully completed the task, as did the President's brother, Robert. And groups of all ages across the country set out to prove to the world that America was as youthful and vigorous as the Kennedy image itself. As it happened, however, this was not the best way to do it. Hundreds upon hundreds gave up with aching limbs and sore feet; others forced themselves to complete the course and collapsed with physical exhaustion. At best, it was an unpleasant experience. The walks were held on

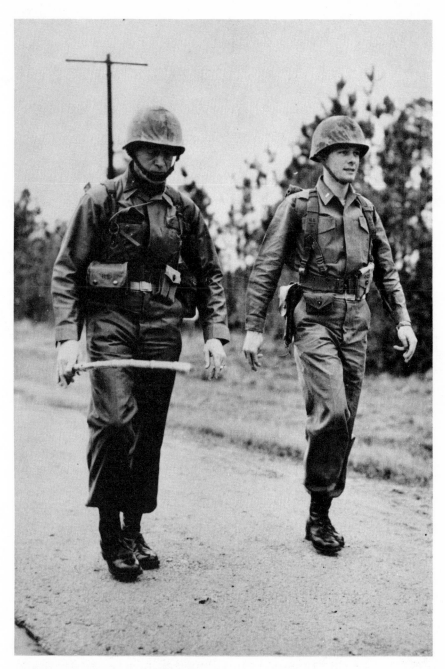

A fifty-year-old Marine Corps veteran, General Rathvon McC.
Tompkins, and a young lieutenant, Charles Bryan, set out on a
fifty-mile hike, following President Kennedy's challenge to complete the
distance as proof of the country's undiminished vigor.

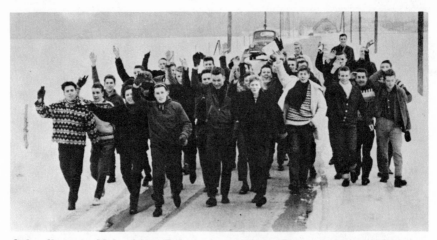

Schoolboys in Nykoebing Falstar in southern Denmark respond to JFK's call to youth. They completed the distance over four consecutive days, with less pain and, no doubt, more benefit than those in the US who tried to squeeze the distance into three or less days, as President Theodore Roosevelt had originally stipulated when he challenged the Marines in 1908.

cordoned-off highways on which participants were oppressed not only by the rigors of walking on concrete for so many miles but also by plain boredom.

To underline the second principle – long-term improvement – you should consider what you are trying to do. You are asking your muscles to strengthen, your heart to beat more strongly, your arteries to open, your ligaments to ease. It takes time to adapt. Don't think in terms of weeks, but in terms of months or even a whole year. That way there will be no formidable barriers that you feel you *must* overcome, no daily grind to dread. *You* make the rules. You can choose both the level you want to reach and the gradient of the slope. Make it a gentle one and the climb will be easy. At the end of a year you'll find your life will have a new and healthier pattern – one you won't want to unravel in a hurry.

Born to Walk

Before you start combining willpower, muscles, sinews and heart in a year-long walk to good health, it may be a help to remember that however unfit you are, your unfitness is in a way superficial. Whatever you lack in the way of fitness, you

*"Few men know how to take a walk. The qualifications . . . are
endurance, plain clothes, old shoes, an eye for Nature, good
humor, vast curiosity, good speech, good silence and nothing
too much."*

Ralph Waldo Emerson, *Notes on Walking*

possess, willy-nilly, the framework of a fine walker, for as a
species we evolved to walk.

The apes from which we are descended were not walkers.
Modern apes, with whom we share a common ancestry, have
short bowed legs and don't like going very far without reverting
to a quadrupedal gait by putting their knuckles on the ground.
Our ancestral relatives broke away from that particular
evolutionary trap. By some five million years ago, there had
evolved man-like creatures that survived by making themselves
relatively independent of trees. These were the Australopithe-
cines of central Africa. With their shambling gait, they were
poor walkers over long distances, but could walk short distances well enough. The first true man – our direct ancestor –
is suitably known as *Homo erectus*, upright man. *Homo erectus*'s
thighbones were tucked into its pelvis in a way that enabled it
to walk for long distances without effort. Its foot was arched to
support its weight efficiently and its toes had lost all traces of
the grasping ability that ape feet still possess.

Some anthropologists believe that the evolution of walking
was the all-important stimulus that impelled our half-ape
ancestors to evolve as they did. An upright gait freed the hands
from the need to act as supporting limbs and allowed the dex-
trous use of tools. This in turn led to the development of an
intelligence to match. Our ability to walk, therefore, made us
what we are as a species. We have inherited a skeletal foundation that will survive almost unscathed a lot more than a few
years of desk work and heavy lunches. Walking is literally in
the framework of our bones.

It may seem strange, therefore, to realize that one can *learn*
to walk better. Mostly, we just walk and there's an end to it. It's
so natural that we normally never stop to analyze it. In fact,
there is a lot to walking.

Let's look at the stride itself. When the heel of the lead foot

> "When people are ill and they come to see you in a hospital, often an aspirin is all they need. But if you prescribe it they sneer at you. They expect something more than an aspirin. I find that to get them to take an aspirin, I have to prescribe something else along with it.
>
> "Walking is like aspirin. It's hard to envision that if we just pick up our pace we're doing something dramatic. But nevertheless walking is your basic prescription for health, more often than not. Unfit people don't need anything else to get them fit."
>
> Dr. John Waller, New York Hospital for Special Surgery

touches the ground, the leg is ever so slightly flexed – the best possible combination of pillar-like strength to catch your weight and a slight give to prevent jarring. By the time the lead foot has rolled onto the ground, the leg is quite straight. As the lead foot lands, it tends to decelerate the body. The acceleration comes from the rear leg, which bows out at the back as the toes thrust it forward. The rear leg then swings through like a pendulum (at low speed it does so almost under its own momentum and requires hardly any energy expenditure at all) to take on its share of support as the leading leg.

At low speeds this is a beautifully relaxed progression but as you begin to stretch out, you'll find it more demanding. This is because as you begin to increase the length of your stride, the rest of the body is brought increasingly strongly into play. The stride is, of course, limited in its length by the length of your legs, but anyone can learn to reach further forward at each pace to increase speed and energy expenditure. You can do this with a conscious swing of the hips. The distance between the top of the thighs is about eight inches. If you can consciously swing your hips as you walk, you can put several inches onto each stride. It doesn't sound like much, but in a long walk, a swinging-hip action that added 4 inches to your stride would cut down the paces you take in a given distance by 250 per mile.

As your pace picks up, you will find other effects occur, all quite natural. In order to counteract the swing in the lower part of your body, your upper part will counter-rotate. Since it's hard and uncomfortable to swing the trunk, the arms take up the task of counteracting the rotation. They will tend to swing in half-circles. At low speeds this is not obvious because the arms swing slowly and are held straight, but at greater speeds, as they begin to contribute to the overall action, you'll find your arms beginning to bend at the elbow until they are held at about 90 degrees, swinging alternately across your chest and round toward the small of your back.

It's this action in the upper body that makes walking such a marvelous exercise, for at higher speeds the pumping action of the arms ensures multiple benefits: not only will your heart beat faster, but almost every muscle of the body comes into play. Clearly, you will gain leg strength. But you will also be exhilarated by the effect in the small of the back, in the shoulders, in the biceps and in the stomach. It is this combination of muscular activity that helps turn unwanted fat into hard muscle.

So from now on ignore the framework. It's what the framework supports and contains – the system of muscle, blood and skin and assorted organs – that is important for our fitness as individuals (rather than as a species). To strengthen this system, you must use it; and not only use it, but use it increasingly hard. In order to achieve the slowly rising graph of fitness mentioned earlier, you must plan to impose a continuous increase in stress upon your body.

The Good Side of Stress

Stress, as we saw in the previous chapter, does not have a good image; psychological and emotional stress, long sustained and undissipated, can indeed undermine one physically. But stress has an equal and opposite significance. Stress – in our case, muscular stress – that is planned for, accepted and so absorbed by the body contributes to its fitness. If planned muscular stress is increased, fitness grows. This is the principle of overload that underlies any training program, whether it's for a patient recuperating from a disease or an Olympic runner. To be truly effective, and to avoid *over*-overloading, you have to plan not only where you're going, but how you're going to get there day by day and week by week.

In this sense, applying stress – or overloading – means fractional increases either in distance, intensity or time, or in all three. To establish a program and to measure your improvement, the requirements are simple:

91

1. You need a few places to walk, both on the level and uphill.
2. You need to make a rough estimate of the distances available.
3. You need a watch with a second hand (I find them easier than digital watches).
4. You need to keep an accurate finger on your own pulse.

In fact, your pulse rate alone will be your guide and mentor. It tells you how hard you have worked, if you have done too much too quickly and if you can afford to go a little faster. Finally, it will act as a basic measure for your steady increase in fitness.

There are a number of things your pulse rate indicates – for instance, the force of the blood flow, which will become stronger as you get fitter; the volume of the artery, which will increase; the regularity of your heart beat, which will even out. It is unlikely that you will be aware of these factors when you are taking your own pulse. There is a fourth factor, however, that will really be obvious to you: frequency. As you become fitter, the frequency of your pulse rate will diminish.

A lower pulse rate, whether you are at rest or at the end of a strenuous uphill walk, is your first aim. From a lower pulse, all other benefits flow. A lower pulse rate means that your heart takes longer to fill. It becomes a more efficient pump. More oxygen gets into the bloodstream. And, as you will see from looking at Appendix 2 in "The Walker's Yellow Pages," those with lower heart beats can sustain a correspondingly higher maximum heart rate. You will be able to undertake more with a greater margin of safety.

The way to a lower heart rate is, paradoxically, to raise it. Like the other muscles that will respond to your walking program, the heart, too, is composed of muscle tissue which becomes stronger with use. In *Total Fitness* Laurence Morehouse compares the heart and its action to a hand wringing out a wet washcloth. The hand and its fingers represent the heart muscles. Squeezing with one finger won't give you a dry washcloth; an out-of-condition heart is not an efficient pump. What training does is to ensure that all the muscles start working to wring the heart of its blood supply at each beat. That is what fitness is all about.

The secret then is to raise your pulse rate. But to what level should you raise it? There are a number of theoretical guidelines that can help you determine what you should be aiming for. Base your estimate on your maximum heart rate, which is often defined as 220 minus your age. If you're fit and 30, your maximum heart rate is 190; if you're 50, it's 170. But unless you are aiming for super-fitness, it is not necessary to achieve your maximum; and if you're unfit, you shouldn't even try to get near it.

If you're training your *heart* (and there are other considerations, as we shall see later on), the figure you will need to know is, aptly enough, your training heart rate. This is the minimum threshold of intensity necessary to improve cardio-respiratory function. If, after testing yourself, you find that you are in a lower category of fitness, you will probably find you can ignore even this figure. *Any* significant increase in heartbeat which does not lead to discomfort, will have a training effect. But if you've been at it a few months, or if you are halfway fit, it is useful to know what your training heartbeat should be.

Determining Your Training Heartbeat

As a rule of thumb, you can calculate it by one of two methods. The first, which takes little account of individual variations in resting heart rate, is to work out your theoretical maximum heartbeat (220 minus your age) and then take 75 percent of that figure as your training heart rate.

Thus, for a 40-year-old:

$220 - 40 = 180$
75 percent of 180 ($.75 \times 180$) = 135

The second method is somewhat more complicated but also more reliable. Figure out your theoretical maximum heartbeat from Appendix 2. Next take your resting heartbeat and subtract it from your theoretical maximum. Take 60 percent of that figure (or multiply by 0.6). Then add your resting heart rate.

For example, for a 40-year-old with a resting heart rate of 70:

$176 - 70 = 106;$
$106 \times 0.6 = 63.6; 63.6 + 70 = 133.6$ (say 134)

As a 40-year-old, if you are to stress your heart sufficiently to make it stronger, you should, in theory, raise your heartbeat to 136.

93

How high should you take your heartbeat in practice? Well that, of course, depends on you and your level of fitness. Medical researchers over the last few years have devoted considerable time trying to devise ways of assessing the safe upper limit for each individual. But most doctors are happy to rely on the patients themselves. Ian Anderson, for instance, advises people to simply remain aware of their own body and listen to what it's telling them. If you feel tired, weak and exhausted, you *are* tired, weak and exhausted. And if your heartbeat is only 120, well, so be it. That is your working maximum. Don't push it.

The Walker's Way to Slow but Steady Weight Loss

Heart rate may be the most significant factor to be taken into account when planning an exercise program, but it is not the only one. The second major factor is the energy cost of your activity. The energy value of food and human output is usually measured in calories (units that reflect the amount of heat released by a material when it is burned). Simply staying alive burns up a certain amount of energy. This is what is known as your basal metabolism. For someone weighing 150 pounds it's about 2,000–2,500 calories a day. As a rule of thumb, you can work out what you burn daily by multiplying your weight in pounds by 15. Since a pound of fat is equivalent to 3,500 calories, you could, by fasting, lose a pound or more every two days. (But don't do it! You'll dehydrate yourself and possibly cause metabolic deficiencies; and the loss will not be permanent.) Even if you don't raise your heartbeat very much, any extra activity you undertake will help your body machine to burn more energy and tick over more efficiently.

The implications of this are extremely important to anyone concerned about their weight. It is often said that exercise in weight reduction is an insignificant factor. In a way, this is true: as you can see by looking at the tables of calorie expenditure for various activities on pages 95 and 96, you would theoretically have to run for five hours in order to lose a pound of fat. Clearly, no unfit person in their right mind would do such a thing.

But what I am advocating here is *not* a plan for rapid weight loss: we're looking at a program stretched over a year or more.

AVERAGE CALORIE EXPENDITURE

Approximate average values for someone weighing 140–150 pounds

ACTIVITY			CALORIES PER: HOUR	½ HOUR	MINUTE
Sleeping (for comparison)			75	38	1.25
Walking *On level*		2.0 mph	180	90	3.00
		3.0 mph	260	130	4.33
		3.5 mph	300	150	5.00
		4.0 mph	350	175	5.83
		4.5 mph	480	240	8.00
		5.3 mph	620	310	10.33
	Upstairs	1.0 mph	195	98	3.25
		2.0 mph	640	320	10.67
	Downstairs	2.0 mph	215	108	3.58
Running		5.5 mph	660	330	11.00
		7.2 mph	720	360	12.00
		8.0 mph	825	413	13.75
		10.0 mph	1140	570	19.00
		11.4 mph	1390	695	23.17
Hiking *20-lb. pack*		2.5 mph	300	150	5.00
		3.0 mph	312	156	5.20
		3.5 mph	380	190	6.33
		4.0 mph	450	225	7.50
	40-lb. pack	1.0 mph	210	105	3.50
		2.0 mph	270	135	4.50
		3.0 mph	348	174	5.80
		4.0 mph	540	270	9.00
Badminton	*Recreational*		350	175	5.83
	Competitive		600	300	10.00
Baseball	(*Except pitcher*)		300	150	5.00
	Pitcher		400	200	6.67
Basketball			608	304	10.13
Bicycling		5.5 mph	240	120	4.00
		9.0 mph	415	208	6.92
		13.0 mph	660	330	11.00
Bowling			270	135	4.50

Calisthenics *Basic level*		200	100	3.33
Intermediate and advanced levels		400	200	6.67
Canoeing	*Leisurely*	230	115	3.83
	4.0 mph	420	210	7.00
Fencing		630	315	10.50
Golf (*no carts*)		300	150	5.00
Horseback riding (*trot*)		415	208	6.92
Mountain climbing		600	300	10.00
Rowing	2.5 mph	300	150	5.00
	3.5 mph	660	330	11.00
	11.0 mph	970	485	16.17
Skating	*Leisurely*	350	175	5.83
	9.0 mph	470	235	7.83
	11.0 mph	640	320	10.67
	13.0 mph	780	390	13.00
Skiing *On level*	3.0 mph	540	270	9.00
	5.0 mph	720	360	12.00
Downhill	Various	300–500	150–250	5.0–8.33
Snowshoeing	2.5 mph	620	310	10.33
Squash		600–800	300–400	10.00–13.33
Swimming *Crawl*	0.7 mph	300	150	5.00
	1.0 mph	420	210	7.00
	1.6 mph	700	350	11.67
	1.9 mph	850	425	14.17
	2.2 mph	1600	800	26.67
Breaststroke	0.7 mph	300	150	5.00
	1.0 mph	410	205	6.83
	1.3 mph	600	300	10.00
Sidestroke	1.0 mph	550	275	9.17
	1.6 mph	1200	600	20.00
Backstroke	0.8 mph	300	150	5.00
	1.0 mph	450	225	7.50
	1.2 mph	540	270	9.00
	1.3 mph	660	330	11.00
	1.6 mph	800	400	13.33
Table tennis		360	180	6.00
Tennis *Recreational*		450	225	7.50
Competitive and singles		600	300	10.00
Volleyball *Recreational*		350	175	5.83
Competitive		600	300	10.00

Weight goes on slowly, and it should be taken off slowly. To quote Pollack, Wilmore and Fox in *Health and Fitness through Physical Activity*:

By increasing the caloric expenditure by 300–500 calories per day, through a properly prescribed physical activity program, it would be possible to lose a pound of fat in 7–12 exercise sessions (i.e., in two weeks to a month). For most people, this would mean . . . a brisk walk for 45–60 minutes. If a modest diet was also followed, weight and fat reduction would occur at an even faster rate.

In other words, a walking program, combined with a reduction of just one buttered slice of bread per day, would result in a total weight loss of 20–30 pounds per year. Although this is only about half a pound a week, a quantity that hardly shows upon most bathroom scales, it is a yearly loss of which most dieters would be proud. Moreover, the chances are that the loss will be permanent, because new habits of exercise will have been established. And, finally, there's a double bonus: all of the lost weight will be fat, but a whole lot more fat will have been converted into muscle. After a year of small, steady increases in your schedule, you will not only have slimmed down, but you'll have changed shape as well.

How Often How Long?

How often should you walk, and for how long? Michael Pollack has a clear-cut reply: a minimum of three times a week, for a minimum of thirty minutes.

His answer was derived from detailed walking experiments done in the early 1970s on the benefits of different levels of exercise combined with the practical demands of daily life. His results are worth quoting at some length. He and his team designed an experiment to train men at either one, three or five days a week at a standard level of exertion for a standard length of time. The subjects' maximum oxygen uptake (which can be equated with pulse rate) improved in direct relation to the frequency of training. The men who followed the three- and five-day-a-week programs also showed significant changes in body weight and fat content (a two-day-a-week program showed improvement in aerobic capacity, but no change in weight or fat levels).

Pollack's work on the intensity and duration of walking necessary for improvement is equally significant. "It is important to reiterate that duration and intensity are interrelated and that the total amount of work (energy cost) accomplished in a training program is the most important factor for fitness development," he wrote. "For example, the energy cost of running is generally higher than walking. Yet many men and women would rather walk than run. Since the intensity of walking is less than running, can one expect to get similar training effects by walking if the duration and frequency are increased?"

He decided to find out with a walking program measuring the performance of sixteen sedentary men 40 to 57 years old over twenty weeks. They walked for about forty minutes, four days per week, at just over 4 MPH. They progressed from 2.5 miles per session in 35.8 minutes (4.26 MPH) to 3.2 miles in 41 minutes (4.74 MPH). The results were startling. The measured improvements as a result of this program were equal to that of a thirty-minute, three-day-per-week jogging program. The subjects' resting heart rates dropped from 65 to 62 beats per minute, and they lost 2 to 3 pounds in weight, all of it fat. The lower intensity of walking was offset by the increased duration and frequency of training – a finding that will surprise many runners, convinced as they are that only by running can they achieve and sustain fitness. It's hard to underestimate the significance of Pollack's findings for the millions of people who prefer *not* to run. By walking more, you can change your lives. You really can.

But the progress was not only a success in physiological terms. It was also a success in social and personal terms. Pollack was working with a small team who came to him as a result of an advertisement in the local paper. They came because they felt themselves to be in need of exercise. But as Pollack told me: "Half of them would not have joined the program at all if they'd had to jog. They admitted they were afraid of it. Most of them knew exercise would be a good thing and thought walking would be a good way to get started. Afterwards, they were delighted. They really enjoyed it."

One of those who took part in the program was Franklin Shirley, a professor in the Speech and Communications Department of Wake Forest University in Winston-Salem, North

Carolina. "I was concerned about my physical well-being," he told me. "I had slightly high blood pressure and was taking a pill a day to control that. It wasn't anything very serious but I knew I wasn't getting anywhere near enough exercise. Pollack's program provided an excellent opportunity. After it, I felt much better. My heartbeat was slower, I was more relaxed and I slept better."

And now? "Well, that was six years ago. I became mayor and gave up regular exercising except for a bit of bike riding. I was working too hard, not getting enough rest. Then last year, I suffered a light stroke. Since then I've taken it easy. But I need to build up. I wish I could do the program again. I'll be incorporating the techniques I learned with Pollack into my new exercise program as soon as I can."

The Basic Program

Now that you know the principles and what you can hope to achieve, let's see what you should be doing in practice. The exercise prescription recommended by Mike Pollack is a three-stage one:

1. A starter program.
2. Slow progression.
3. Maintenance.

The purpose of the starter program is to start you exercising at a low level, well within the capacity of even the unfittest. The low-level start is important. It allows the body time to adapt properly so that there is no soreness in the muscles or discomfort in the knees or feet, and also it allows you to improve quickly.

The last point is a vital one. Usually in the first weeks, you will not experience much change in weight. The muscles adapt, fat begins to turn into muscle and you may eat a little more to compensate for your increased energy expenditure. But if you are hoping for encouragement from the bathroom scales, you may be disappointed. The only way to measure your progress is by your increasing ability to walk farther and faster. That's encouraging.

Stage 1: The Starter Program
The starter program usually lasts four to six weeks, but the time

depends on your level of fitness and your age. As a guide, it takes 40 percent longer for each decade in life after 30 to adapt to a new physical regime. A starter program that takes four weeks for a 30-year-old, should be stretched out to seven weeks for a 65-year-old.

In Appendix 3 of "The Walker's Yellow Pages" you will find a starter program based on a routine recommended by Mike Pollack. It is simplified in that it involves only your body, a flat surface (a street, a field or a track), a watch and an ability to count your paces so you know how fast you're going.

A few words on this last item are in order. It's extremely difficult to work out walking speed accurately, but don't despair: there's a rough-and-ready relationship between miles-per-hour and paces-per-minute. Although obviously a short person has a shorter stride and tends to walk slower and vice versa for a tall person, you can still estimate your speed by remembering that 120 paces a minute, or 2 paces every second, is equivalent to 4 MPH (assuming a pace of one yard). You don't even need a watch to establish this rhythm. 120 paces a minute is military marching speed. As you walk, if you hum the *British Grenadiers*,

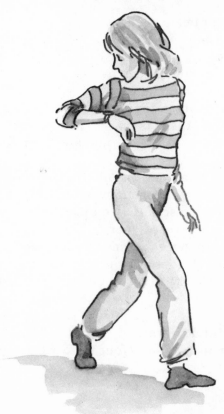

"I have been taking daily walks for some thirty years and I conclude that, though habit-forming, the practice is not quickly fatal."

John Kieran, *A Spring Walk*

Colonel Bogey or whatever (depending on your national allegiance) and keep pace with the beat, you'll be walking at about 4 MPH. It's equally easy to estimate half that speed – one pace per second – but it will almost certainly be too slow to be of any interest to you, unless you're climbing a steep hill.

When walking faster or slower, the easiest way to establish a rhythm is to count your paces over 10 or 15 seconds. Once established, you will find it quite easy to distinguish a 3 MPH pace, say, from 3.5 MPH. A speed of 3 MPH is 88 paces per minute, which is 22 paces in 15 seconds. 3.5 MPH is 26 paces in 15 seconds – an increase significant enough to establish a new rhythm.

Some words of warning: This should be an easy program. You don't have to drive yourself to exhaustion:

1. If you feel tired, stop. Take your pulse. After ten minutes' rest, if your heart is still over 100 beats per minute, take things more slowly.

2. Don't impose extra, unnecessary strains on your system by walking in great heat or cold. Ideally, you should walk within a 40–85° F temperature range, with humidity less than 60 percent.

3. Don't stand still or sit motionless after exercising. Rest by all means, but move your limbs about to ensure good circulation as your heart rate returns to normal.

After a week or two, you'll be able to see a measurable improvement in your performance: you'll be walking further and faster with a lower heart rate. But you should also be receiving feedback in other ways. In Dr. Fox's words, new walkers "feel they have more energy and interest. They sparkle more. They feel more creative and enthusiastic. They can sit through tedious committee meetings without losing concentration."

The starter program will involve you in less than half an hour three times a week, but in the course of those six weeks, you will have covered thirty-six miles on foot and expended over three thousand calories. If you've cut down a bit on your diet you may even have lost a few pounds. You'll certainly be stronger. If you're more than twenty or thirty pounds overweight, a measurable amount of fat will have turned to muscle. You'll have greater confidence in your own physical capacity. All of which makes a good return on a very small investment of effort.

Don't worry that the calorie cost is still rather low in the starter program; you have to give your body time to adapt. If you're a rank beginner and very unfit, you'll be in the same position as my 260-pound cab driver Leonard Kommissar, who, when I met him, had been walking for only a few days. "In the morning, I wake up, drive over to Central Park and park at a cab stand. All I'm doing right now is walking from 61st to 66th Street and back, about ten blocks, half a mile. I'm not in any rush, I'm not trying to beat no clocks, I figure it'll take eight, nine months, a year, to get fit. Steady progress." Right on, Mr. K.

Stage 2: Slow Progression
Once you've been through the starter program, you'll want to move on to the next stage of slow progression. You'll see that this second program takes you from a speed of about 4 MPH on the level up to a speed of 6 MPH. For walking this is a tremendous speed. If you can manage this speed, you may well prefer to progress to a running program. If running isn't for you, though, there is another way of achieving the same level of energy consumption – by walking uphill. It has been shown that walking at 4 MPH up a 15 percent gradient (1:6) is equivalent to running at 8 MPH on the flat. If you're not used to running and don't want to do it, you'll find that you'll get far more benefit and enjoyment from walking uphill. It will seem natural to you and you'll run no risk of injury. But your pulse rate will be way up – as it should be – and you'll be using all the muscles that you would be using if you were running.

Tricks of the Trade
I've just asked you to consider a program that is, above all, very

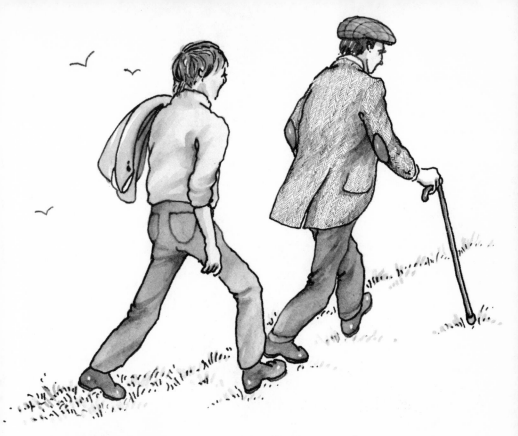

regular. In fact, as we all know, life is not always so easy. Perhaps you're extra busy; perhaps you have relatives or friends staying with you; perhaps the weather turns against you; perhaps you get ill. There are any number of reasons why you might miss a day here and there, even with the best will in the world. Whatever you do, don't give up. There are some tricks you should be aware of that can be used either to fill in the gaps or to extend the program you're already following. They are based on the fact that any activity involves energy expenditure. Whether you are doing housework or walking to work or going up stairs, you are still taking some form of exercise. It is quite possible to formalize many of the activities that you perform almost unconsciously every day and build them into your fitness program.

Take housework for instance. If you weigh 150 pounds, you use up about 270 calories an hour making beds, which is about 175 calories above your hourly basal metabolism. Walking up stairs at 2 MPH (say two steps per second) uses double the energy that walking on the level does at 4 MPH. Half the speed, double the energy.

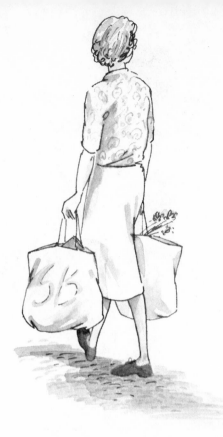

Indeed it's quite possible to get fit simply by walking up stairs. In a fitness campaign conducted by the London *Sunday Times* in 1976, a 57-year-old-housewife, Sylvia Baynham, did just this. "I chose this method of exercise because I hate the cold," she said, "and the thought of going for a walk or a run in the winter just meant I would never exercise. Now I can exercise whenever I have fifteen minutes to spare. No changing into special clothes, no driving to a swimming pool or a sports center; just shoes off and up and down those stairs."

Her routine involved choosing a flight of ten stairs and going up and down them at the rate of five times a minute. This is not much of a problem for just one minute, but it is extremely demanding to do so fifty times in ten minutes. "People have asked me if I get bored and what I think about. In fact, I don't have much time to think, I'm too busy counting my trips. And as to being bored, well surely, if it is boring, it's worth it for such a short time to get fit."

But you do not have to be as formal about it as Sylvia Baynham. It would come as a surprise to most housewives just how much exercise they do get every day simply as part of their routine and how little extra they need to build a very sound level of fitness. It's the same with office workers and commuters. J. N. Morris's famous study of 17,000 London civil servants found a significant difference in fitness between those who had to walk the odd half mile to or from the train station and those who didn't.

It is not hard to look upon a necessary daily walk as an opportunity. A half-mile walk at either end of a working day is an extra five miles a week. If your route involves going up an escalator, use this as an opportunity as well. Don't simply stand on the escalator. Walk up it. Even moving at an average pace (allowing for rush hour crowds, of course), you can cover the equivalent of half its length before you arrive at the top. Those twenty or thirty steps count toward your energy expenditure. When you emerge from the station to walk the half mile to the office, stretch out a little. Time yourself over a set distance. Count your number of paces per minute. Then, week by week, increase your pace per minute and decrease the time it takes you to cover the distance. In a few months you'll find you'll be able to risk leaving the office a little later and still make the train without collapsing in a sweaty heap into the nearest seat.

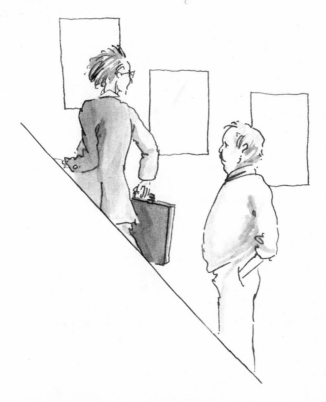

"Time is not money; time is an opportunity to live before you die. So a man who walks, and lives and sees and thinks as he walks, has lengthened his life."

Donald Culross Peattie, *The Joy of Walking*

This approach is increasingly recommended by doctors. For instance, Dr. Irving S. Wright, Emeritus Clinical Professor of Medicine at Cornell, was recently quoted in *The Jogger* magazine as saying, "I tell my patients to get off the subway a station or two early and walk the rest of the way." Dr. Wright himself often makes a point of walking down fifteen flights of stairs from his office in New York Hospital.

Again, as Dr. Fox told me in Washington, "Walking is clearly appropriate for an individual who has been riding in his own automobile or taking public transportation and doing very little walking and very little stair climbing, who always tries to find the parking spot exactly next to the entrance of whatever building he is visiting. This individual can do a great deal to get started with a valuable reconditioning effort by not looking for the closest parking spot, but actually looking for a parking spot that gives him an opportunity to walk, and to avoid taking the elevators where the stairwells are attractive and safe. . . ."

There is one activity normally regarded as sporting which it is extremely easy to make more energetic: golf. Whatever else golf is, the actual business of hitting a ball provides hardly any exercise. In 1965 a young medic named Leroy Getchell published the results of a study he'd undertaken on the physical effects of golf. He found that golfers showed no increase in strength or agility as a result of swinging their woods and irons. But the study did reveal that there were hidden benefits from playing golf – benefits that had nothing to do with the accuracy or power of the strokes. They derived from the golfer's need to walk for several miles.

About one-third of the time on a golf course is spent walking (unless, of course, you ride from hole to hole in a golf cart, in which case there will be no measurable physical benefits). The golfers in Getchell's study – twenty of them – were amateurs from the Urbana, Illinois, area, who averaged just over twelve hours of play per week from April to September. He found that after a season of golf (or walking, whichever way you like to look at it) the players' maximum heart rates, as measured on a treadmill, were significantly reduced from an average of 163.8 to 157. In eighteen holes of golf, each golfer burned up a not inconsiderable 1,000 calories.

In another study, a doctoral dissertation done for Oklahoma State University in 1969, Bernard Crowell found that when golfers were carrying their own clubs, they developed an average heartbeat of 113 beats per minute. The lessons are obvious: if you walk the course and carry your own clubs, and if you walk as fast as is compatible with a steady swing and a retention of concentration on the putting green, you can make quite a significant contribution to your walking program *and* to your growing fitness.

Stage 3: Maintenance

At the end of twenty-six weeks if you are 30 – or after almost a year if you're 50 (remember, you should be stretching the program by 40 percent for every decade of your age) – you will have achieved, through walking, a level of fitness of which you can justifiably be proud.

You will probably now be hooked on the need to walk several times a week. So much the better. Fitness is not stored; it has to be preserved by continuous activity. You now have the best of all possible choices: you can simply continue your program or you can develop it in any number of ways. If you want to continue walking, take whatever tips you can from other chapters in this book. Invite friends who know about your town or city or the surrounding countryside to walk with you. Take day walks with groups or by yourself. Climb hills. Alternatively, you may want to become involved in other athletic activities and you can now do so in perfect safety.

Your basic walking program will have lasted anything from six months to a year. But the actual time spent walking need be no more than 120 hours – a total of no more than five days in all. If you care to work it out, you'll find that this is a mere 0.0002 percent of your life expectancy. Yet for that minute investment of time, you will have evolved a new attitude, new and healthier habits and a fitter body. Has anyone ever made you a better deal?

Special Problems

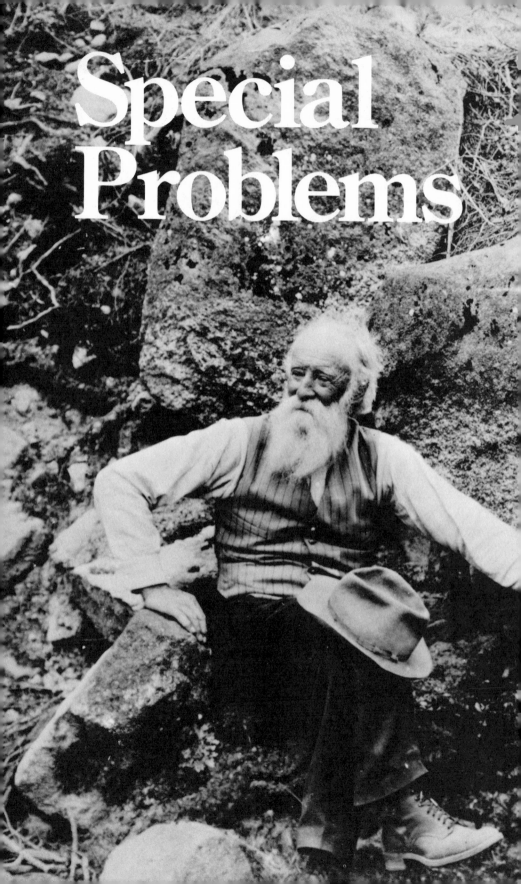

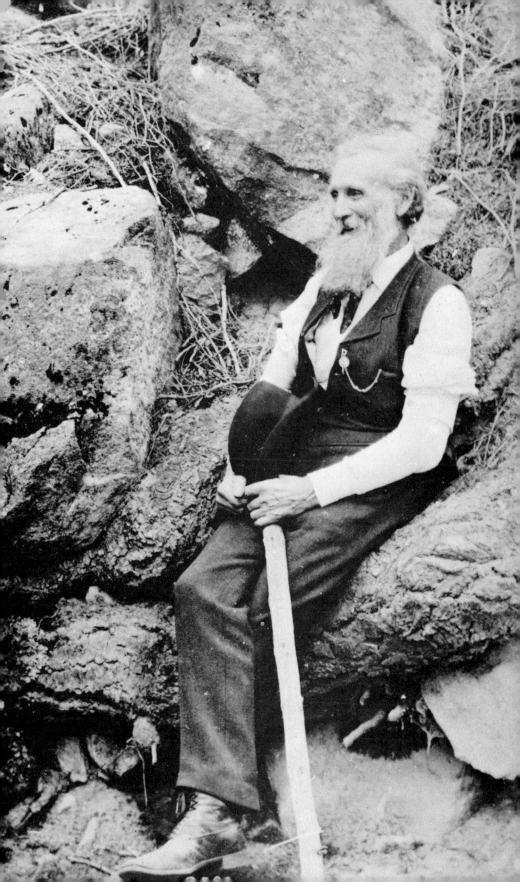

Special Problems

ONE OF OUR MOST basic rights is the right to good health, and it is when our health is most at risk that walking truly comes into its own. This chapter is concerned with three special problem areas, at least one of which will involve everyone sooner or later. They are obesity, old age and recuperation from a heart attack.

Obesity

You will find a certain amount about the problems of being overweight and the advantages of walking in dealing with it in other chapters, but it is such a consuming interest – literally and figuratively – to so many people that the causes and solutions are worth going into in more detail.

It is hard, indeed, to overstate the significance of obesity to the onset of disease. We have already looked at some of the major statistical hazards of being overweight – particularly the chances of dying younger and the strain imposed on bones, muscles and heart. The list of associated complaints is truly formidable. Since the heart has to push the blood through miles of extra capillaries, obesity not only places a greater strain on the heart, but leads to increased blood pressure. The obese have trouble breathing normally and have a greater incidence of respiratory infections. Since their circulatory systems are less efficient, they tend to have more carbon-dioxide and less oxygen in their blood, and therefore have a tendency to be lethargic. Gall bladder disease, degenerative arthritis, diabetes, gout and even cancer are statistically related to obesity. And it is also tragically true that because many obese individuals are unhappy with their appearance and with their inability to control their own weight they may be under continual emotional stress. To quote Dr. Edgar Gordon in *The Physician and Sportsmedicine* journal. "If you take all these things together, you realize that this constellation of clinical conditions is the most important group of problems that the medical profession has to face."

There are four major causes of putting on weight: a hereditary tendency; overeating; sedentary living; and psychological problems – all four of which are interrelated to a certain extent. But whatever the cause of your weight problem – whether you're fifteen or fifty pounds overweight – I'm sure you can find something of use here.

Unless you are one of those rare medical cases in which metabolism is so severely affected that it results in obesity, for almost all of you who are overweight, the basic problem is a social one. Western society has institutionalized the ingestion of at least three meals a day, with countless other accepted opportunities throughout the day for "light refreshments" – mid-morning coffee breaks; mid-afternoon tea; drinks around 6 o'clock served up with peanuts, potato chips, crackers and cheese, and the like, the proverbial midnight snack, and so on. Often these are considered as "snacks" rather than full meals, and as such can happily be ignored. But in terms of a calorific intake, they can easily be the equivalent of a meal. A couple of martinis and a few handfuls of peanuts comes to five hundred calories – more than most people typically eat for breakfast.

The social pressures to indulge come from friends and colleagues and are hard to refuse – "Go on, Charlie, have another beer, it won't do you any harm." "Just finish up this little slice of chocolate cake, dear. It's only a mouthful and it won't keep till tomorrow." The issue is so small that it seems hardly worth resisting – or offending the offering friend.

Some people don't need to resist. I once had a farming friend who drank two pints of beer at lunch and another two in the evenings in addition to eating three hearty meals, yet he always looked as though he was about to succumb to starvation. Others definitely do need to resist. Some are born with a hereditary tendency to put on fat – not in the sense that they will automatically become fat, but because they burn a given amount of food at a slower speed. This could be a physiological advantage: such people get more mileage from the same amount of fuel and therefore have a more efficient body chemistry. They could survive quite happily on one meal a day, but it would seem antisocial to do so, and it would go against the long-ingrained habits of childhood. The result is that from early adulthood, they eat more than they need – less perhaps than other people, but still more than they *need* – and the pounds continue to mount up.

Another theory which has received a good deal of attention since it was proposed in the early 1970s is that adults become obese because they have a tendency toward obesity built into them as children. A growing child builds fat cells along with the rest of his body, and in children who overeat the body may respond to the excess of food not simply by expanding the cells available, but by building more cells. An average adult complement of fat cells is 25–30 billion; a fat child may grow into an adult with a 100 billion fat cells. Clearly, the adult with three times as many fat cells may always have a problem in preserving a healthy weight.

This theory is by no means proven, but whatever the truth it has been statistically established that fat parents tend to have fat children. This fact is not necessarily due to either a hereditary tendency toward fatness or to the creation of extra fat cells in childhood. One usually needs to look no further than the eating habits of the family. Fat parents encourage their children to eat what they consider a "normal" amount of food. Even if they discourage eating between meals, children will grow up eating, entirely unconsciously, more than they really need. For some people, breakfast is not breakfast without bacon and eggs, a couple of pieces of toast with butter and marmalade, and two cups of coffee, each with three lumps of sugar. Supper is not complete unless there is dessert.

I once got into the habit of eating executive lunches myself. After a year or two of expense-account eating, the hunger pangs around half past twelve were so intense that I couldn't deny to myself that I was hungry. I *had* to eat. As a result, I began to put on weight. Not much – perhaps an average of

"The land of our better selves is most surely reached by walking."

Dr. John Huston Finley

three or four pounds a year, which fortunately tended to evaporate again on holiday and over the summer when I used to
exercise more. When I eventually broke the habit, I realized
that I felt hungry because I was used to having lunch at that
time, not because my body genuinely needed food. I hate to
think what I'd look like now if I'd gone on that way.

For women, the problem is infinitely more complex. As
Susie Orbach has pointed out in *Fat Is a Feminist Issue*, women
may find themselves confronted by pressures that combine to
drive them toward fatness, however much they think they want
to be thin. Certainly, the pressures on women to combine a
variety of roles – wife, mother, homemaker, lover, career
woman – impose on them conflicting demands that men do not
have to face. One response may be to seek reassurance by
eating, an activity considered by many psychologists to be
reassuring because it connects with the basic nurturing role for
which women are biologically fitted.

It's certainly common experience that depression and overeating react upon each other: "When I feel depressed, I eat.
When I eat, I put on weight. When I put on weight, I get depressed. When I'm depressed, I eat. . . ." It's a cycle that most
women (though few men) face at least some time during their
lives.

Most women, at some time, try and break the social and
emotional constraints by dieting. This, on its own, may be
extremely hard to do in the long term. For one thing, it may
mean fighting the habits of years. For another, it means
fighting social pressures. And thirdly, it may mean coming
to grips with the psychological pressures that are driving them
toward fatness in the first place. The effort is bound to be
emotionally demanding. It is also pretty well bound to be
unsuccessful in that unless the woman accomplishes a complete
change in herself and her eating habits, she will relax again
into the pattern that made her fat in the first place. The result
is that countless women with a tendency toward fatness go
through life with a nagging sense of failure, that they can't live
up to the expectations of others, that they can't assert themselves as individuals and that they can't even control themselves sufficiently to stop eating.

For most women the binge-diet seesaw is an unsatisfactory
way of life. What they are seeking is a physical and psychologi-

cal balance. To achieve it by dieting alone is very unusual. But I believe it would help countless women if, instead of seeking to balance two inconsistent elements – their weight and their emotional reaction to it – they added another element to the equation: a walking program.

Walking does three things that dieting on its own can never do, especially if you walk instead of eat:

1. It uses up energy in a positive way. You are doing something active instead of eating, and temptation is easier to resist.

2. It makes you physically healthier by reducing fat and adding lean weight at the same time, and

3. It actually suppresses hunger pangs, thus making it easier to stick to your diet.

If you look at the alternatives, you'll see that there are just three basic ways to lose weight. You can take in less energy by dieting; you can use up more energy by doing more exercise; or you can combine the two approaches.

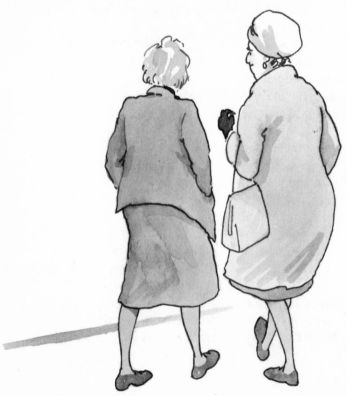

Dieting by itself, as we have seen, has its limitations. You need on average about 2,500 calories per day to keep your body ticking over, and if you take in much less than that, not only do you feel hungry, but you also risk failing to provide yourself with adequate nutrition. If you do a heavy amount of exercise and keep up the same eating habits, you can certainly lose weight and you'll certainly be healthier. But it's hard work. A more commonsense approach is to combine the two techniques: cut down on your calorie intake slightly while at the same time embarking on a moderate program of exercise.

A study conducted by Drs. W. B. Zuti and L. A. Golding and reported in *The Physician and Sportsmedicine* journal in January 1976 quantified the beneficial effects of walking in weight loss by comparing these varying approaches. The study concentrated on basic principles and its results are therefore equally applicable to men and to women.

Drs. Zuti and Golding gathered twenty-five women between 25 and 42 who were anything from twenty to forty pounds overweight and eager to undertake a sixteen-week study. For three weeks before the program, all the women recorded their eating habits meticulously to determine their average calorie intake. They were then divided into three groups. The women in the first group cut back their daily intake by 500 calories. The second group ate the same amount as usual, but took exercise that created a 500-calorie deficit per day. The women in the third group each reduced their daily intake by 250 calories, and increased their energy expenditure by 250 calories. The exercisers worked out for no more than one hour a day, five days a week, on a treadmill.

At the end of sixteen weeks, the women were weighed and measured. They had all lost weight, and the weight loss was roughly the same for each group – between 10.6 and 12 pounds. But the really significant difference was in the relationship between body fat and lean tissue. The dieters, on average, lost 9.5 pounds of body fat and 2.5 pounds of lean tissue. Those in the two exercise groups (the difference between them was not statistically significant) lost 12.5 pounds of body fat, but *gained* between 1 and 2 pounds in lean tissue.

The conclusion is clear cut: at the end of just sixteen weeks of a moderate walking program, you will not only be twelve pounds lighter, but you will be leaner, fitter and firmer. And

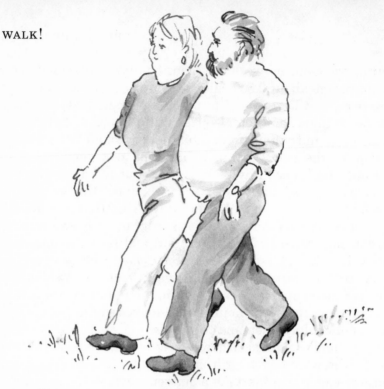

you will have a surer foundation for continued exercising. Even
if you revert to your previous eating habits, the chances are
that as long as you keep walking to ensure a good energy
balance your weight loss will be permanent.

The really startling thing about Drs. Zuti and Golding's
findings is the very small change in the calorie balance involved. A deficit of 250 calories is the equivalent of a forty-five
minute walk at 4 miles an hour on the level. 500 calories is the
equivalent of a $1\frac{1}{2}$-hour's walk, which admittedly is a lot to use
up in exercise on a daily basis. But even if you lose 500 calories
a week (which you can do by walking on average just an extra
fifteen minutes a day), you could reckon on losing a pound in
seven weeks, or seven pounds a year – assuming, of course, that
you keep your intake the same as it was when you begin.

This is the non-diet way to lose weight: it cannot fail. More-
over dieting and exercise mutually reinforce each other. It's
often assumed that taking more exercise affects the appetite.
"What's the use of exercise?" you sometimes hear people say.
"It only makes you eat more." Not so. A 1972 study by Dr.
Merle Foss, associate professor and director of the Physical
Performance Research Laboratory at the University of Michi-
gan, Ann Arbor, showed that unaccustomed exercise – his

subjects were men who were asked to run no more than a mile –
made no measurable difference to the amount of food they con-
sumed over the next twenty-four hours. Even an hour's vigorous
exercise a day does not increase appetite. To do that, you have
to take long hours of physical labor; lumberjacks working
eight to ten hours a day do consume more food. Paradoxically,
short bouts of exercise have exactly the opposite effect. Not
only do you miss a meal, but you don't feel hungry either.

If you're very fat, there's no reason why you shouldn't begin
the basic walking program, but there are a number of problems
you may encounter. The first is a build-up of heat. A fat person's
surface area is less in proportion to his or her body volume. In
other words, the bigger you are the more there is of you on the
inside and the longer it takes for heat to radiate away. This
needn't affect you if you avoid walking on a very hot day. A
second problem is related to breathing. Sometimes the dia-
phragm is constricted in fat people and they have trouble in
taking a deep breath. Or they may experience listlessness caused
by the retention of carbon-dioxide. If you find this happening, it
means that you'll have to take it very easily. Thirdly, you may
encounter some basic mechanical difficulties – muscle soreness
or ankle pains, for instance. Once again the only thing to do is
find your own level.

A Ripe Old Age

The chances are that most people will live *well* beyond their
retirement age. In the West men have a life expectancy of about
70 and women of about 75. If you are now over 45, though,
you can expect to live until you're 72 if you're a man and 78 if
you're a woman. Moreover, you won't be alone when you reach
retirement age: 14 percent of the population of the UK and
20 percent of the USA are over 65. So, theoretically, you could
have time and companionship enough to establish new careers
and indulge long-forgotten interests.

Theoretically. But in practice the problems of aging are
intense. Feelings of depression, rejection and loneliness are
often overwhelming. I remember once talking to an extraordinarily fit-looking elderly man at a lunch party – I took him
for perhaps 65 or 70. He was wearing a tweed coat and had a
military bearing. We got talking about the events he had ex-

"A walk in the woods . . . is one of the secrets for dodging old age."

Ralph Waldo Emerson, *Notes on Walking*

---

perienced, and he spoke knowingly of the First World War.

"Were you in it?" I asked.

"Yes," he said, "after all, I am 83."

"Good Lord," I said. "How does it feel?"

"Lonely," he replied. "But then, I've been lonely since 1917."

A special case perhaps, but indicative.

The physical disabilities of age are obvious as well. There is the inevitable decline of strength, flexibility and acuity in the senses – a decline which is all too often accentuated by emotional and physical passivity. It is still possible, however, to maximize the many physical capacities that do remain. Undoubtedly one of the best and most effective ways to achieve a youthful old age is to walk.

Why should one try? Does an active old age increase longevity? The studies so far are somewhat equivocal. Even those who advocate intensive running programs through life do not claim that running actually makes you live longer. Dr. Thomas Bassler – whose claim that marathoning gives immunity to heart attacks has earned him a certain fame – ascribes the effects he observes as much to the life style a person adopts as to the exercise itself. It is hard to be a marathoner if you smoke and overeat.

There are two other ways of looking at it.

One is to see that exercise removes those elements from your life that could otherwise shorten it. The relationship between exercise and a full life span was clearly established by a study done in 1965 by Dr. Charles Rose in Boston. Dr. Rose and his team conducted extensive and detailed interviews with the next of kin of five hundred men who had died in the city that year. Taking into account some two hundred factors, Dr. Rose found that the best indicator of a future old age was the amount of leisure hours people spent on physical exertion, particularly during their 40s. This, of course, means a long-term commitment to exercise. But if you're already 65 and have long been out of the habit of exercising, don't lose heart. It has been

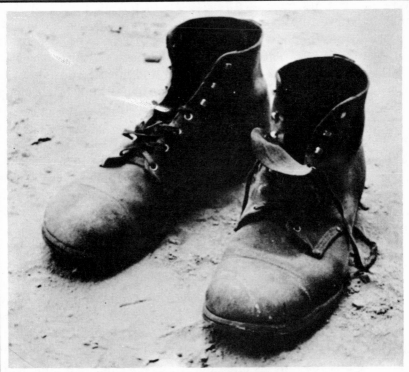

Burroughs's walking boots—rugged but not overheavy, and molded by thousands of miles of tramping to the shape of his feet.

These Boots Were Made for Walking

John Burroughs and John Muir, two of America's greatest naturalists and walkers, were both over 70 when the classic photograph on pp. 108–9 was taken of them in 1910.

Burroughs *(left)* was an Easterner – a memorial to him stands at the summit of Slide Mountain in the Catskills – but he also wandered through Alaska and over the Rockies, camping out with Muir and President Theodore Roosevelt.

John Muir, a Scotsman by birth, is best known as the prime mover in the establishment of Yosemite National Park and other wilderness areas (one of which is named after him). Muir believed that in walking the wilderness, man could find salvation. "Climb the mountains," he wrote, "and get their good tidings. Nature's peace will flow into you as sunshine flows into trees." He once climbed to the top of a 100-foot pine in the midst of a gale to hear the song of the wind in the needles. On another occasion he leaped from his cabin during a violent tremor, shouting ecstatically, "A noble earthquake! A noble earthquake!" His fascination with the wilderness and his apparently endless energy lent him an aura of youthfulness, even in old age.

shown that walking and other forms of physical activity can slow – and even halt – physical decline. Heart and muscles can still be strengthened – not simply stabilized – with use until well into the 70s. The benefits are no less telling – even if less in absolute terms – than in youth and middle age. There is an inevitable decline in later years, but it need not be as steep and dramatic as is usually assumed. There are 70-year-olds who have completed the Boston Marathon. Age is no barrier to an active life style.

The classic case of the rejuvenating power of exercise concerns a Santa Monica grandmother, Eula Weaver, who began an exercise and diet program with the Longevity Research Institute in Santa Barbara, California. When she began at the age of 81, with high blood pressure and degenerative changes in the heart and joints, she could walk no more than a hundred feet and had such bad circulation that she had to wear gloves, even in summer. By 1978, at the age of 88, she was running a mile each morning and was also working out on a stationary bicycle. Eula Weaver may be an exceptional case but she is living proof that the apparent effects of old age can be beaten. There may not be very much that you can do about the years on your life, but you can, as one doctor put it to me, do a good deal to improve the life in your years.

If, in old age, you are not used to walking very much, there's no reason why you can't begin at the beginning of the basic walking program and see how much you can do with comfort. Then build up slowly at your own rate. If you find a single session a bit tough, you can always divide it up into several daily sessions of a few minutes each. This way the muscles will adapt more easily to the tasks you ask them to undertake. In the words of Mike Pollack, "The older individual may need to start the exercise program at a much lower level and progress at a slower rate, but given time the benefits will be the same."

If you are already quite active, you may do better to choose the level at which you feel most comfortable and stick to it, deriving from your walks the pleasure in people and places I cover in other chapters.

One with special knowledge of the benefits of walking in old age, and of the ailments old age brings, is 77-year-old Alfred G. ("Bob") Roberts, a retired sports journalist and a leading light

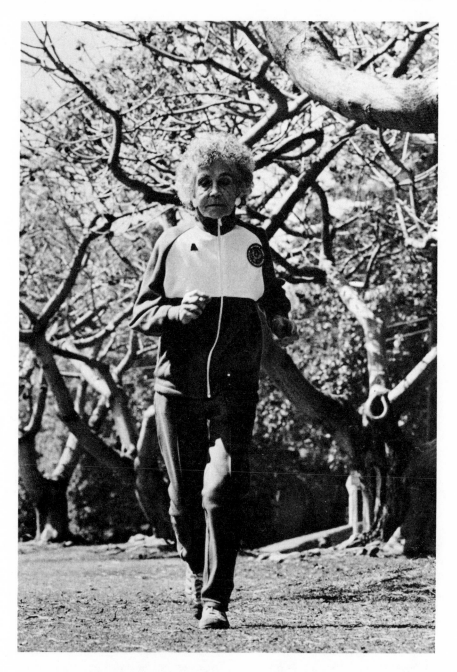

At 88, Eula Weaver is living proof that the effects of old age can often be reversed. At 78, she was crippled by arthritis and the effects of a stroke; she now runs a mile a day, goes to the gym three times a week and pedals ten miles a day on a stationary bicycle.

121

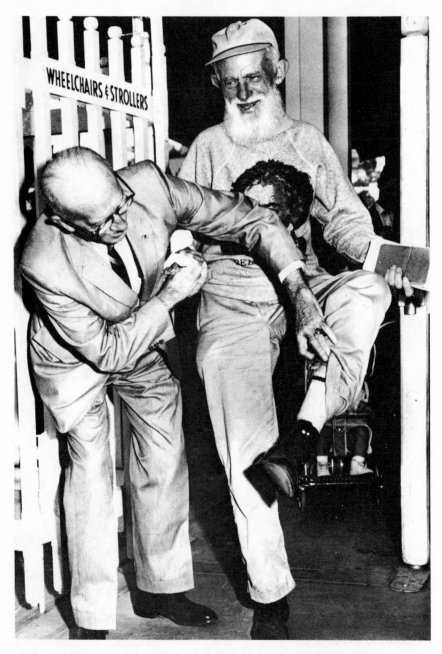

A Seattle World's Fair official examines the legs of John Stahl, 80, a retired postal worker who walked to the fair from San Francisco—a distance of 900 miles. "Old Iron Legs," as he's called, got his nickname some twenty-two years previously after completing a 3,500-mile walk when he was 58.

in the movement to formalize competitive athletics for the over-40s (although there's been a Veterans Athletic Club in England since 1931, international veterans championships – or Master's Championships, as they are known in the US – have only been established within the last ten years). Anyone who fears age and infirmity can draw inspiration from Bob's career.

In his youth Bob Roberts was a keen, if mediocre runner. In his 30s he let things slide. In 1945, when he was in his 40s, Bob realized that he was a "rather uncomfortable" two hundred pounds. He turned again to running and helped re-form the Veterans Athletic Club after the war. One day he was persuaded to enter a one-mile novice track walk. To his (and others') surprise, he won easily. He has been walking ever since.

His competitive career was sporadic, but, in his own words, "I always looked with pleasure to my retirement at 65, when I hoped to engage in a full program of events. Then, in 1966, a few months before I was due to retire, I received a really shattering blow: I developed arthritis. I found myself unable to bend my legs, hardly able to sit down, unable to put my socks on or tie my shoelaces. I explained to the doctor that I was a walker and had been competing quite recently. I was told that my training had kept the arthritis at bay, but – and this was the really shattering part – 'You will not race again.'"

But Bob did race again and, despite repeated setbacks, he continues to do so. He described to me how he confounded his doctors and went on to set world records in International Masters Championships. First came a series of exercises to ease his joints. "After a few weeks I was feeling considerably better and more mobile, and when I was discharged the consultant told me I could walk as far as I liked. Whether he realized it was speed walking I indulged in I don't know, but, heartily bucked, I took him at his word and gradually I found less and less difficulty in getting around. I began to race again.

"I felt if I could only keep on walking, there was no reason why I should not be found promenading round the world a hundred years hence as well as I am to-day."

A. N. Cooper, *On the Road to Rome*

"A big disappointment was a Race Walking Association rule that debars a person of 60 or over from competing in national championships. Veteran walkers resent this ruling and argue that an entry should be judged on performance and not age. I can, however, walk in 'open' races and in my county championship. Possibly I am the only man over 70 to have won a county medal: I was in the Highgate Harriers team that won the Middlesex 10-mile championship in 1974."

What physical benefits has he gained by walking? "I have been plagued with accidents," he says wryly, "but in every case I have not only surmounted them but gone on to win honors. A slipped disc threatened to prevent me participating in my first international in 1972, a 15-mile race at London's Crystal Palace. For weeks before the meeting, I was strapped up in a special corset. I was then 70; despite my restricted training, I not only finished first in my over-60s group, but beat many others competing in the 40-60-year-old section.

"Then, in 1975, a few weeks before the USA Masters Championships in White Plains, New York, and the biannual World Masters Championships in Toronto, I blacked out on a staircase in my home and fell over the bannisters to the floor below."

Amazingly, the accident only seemed to make him more determined. "A few days in the hospital followed, but there was not much wrong with me that anyone could see. On my discharge, I resumed training. But when I attempted fast walking, I was immediately conscious of a damaged ham string. More treatment. Improvement again. I felt confident of doing well in the 5,000-meter track walks at White Plains and Toronto, but decided that I would also tackle the 25-kilometer road race in Canada and hope for the best."

Despite injuries, he was an easy winner of both 5,000-meter races. In Toronto his time was 28 minutes 9 seconds. In a field of forty, comprising groups 55–59, 60–64, 65–69 and 70+, he actually finished seventh overall. In the 25-kilometer road walk, he won his age group (70+) with a time of 2 hours 37 minutes 55.6 seconds. An old friend of his, Augustus (Gus) Theobald of Australia, was second with a time of 2 hours 48 minutes 53.4 seconds. "I was especially glad to see Gus again," he remembered. "He was 78, but still walking well. Another amazing athlete was Fritz Schreiber of Sweden who, although well over 80, still combines running and walking."

Bob immediately began looking ahead to the 1977 games, to be held in Gothenburg, Sweden. Competition would be tougher: there would be 2,670 competitors from nearly fifty nations. Age groups of 75–79 and 80+ were to be included for the first time.

"But just before Christmas 1976," continued Bob, "arthritis struck again. It seemed to be everywhere. I couldn't sit comfortably, I could hardly get one leg in front of the other. Doctors insist there is no cure for arthritis, but after two or three months of blood tests and tablets it gradually eased. In addition, however, I developed severe prostate trouble, from which I have suffered mildly over recent years.

"It was decided a prostectomy was necessary. With the usual long hospital waiting list a considerable delay seemed inevitable. I thought I'd never be fit for Gothenburg. However, I explained my World Championships commitments and hopes to the consultant and my operation duly took place in mid-April. A prostectomy is a major operation and I was in my seventy-sixth year. Afterwards, I tried light training with a 10-mile walk, but I had a slight hemorrhage so decided that I would train for the 5,000 meters on the track and simply trust to luck in the 20 kilometers when the time came."

He won both the 5,000-meter and 20-kilometer races, again

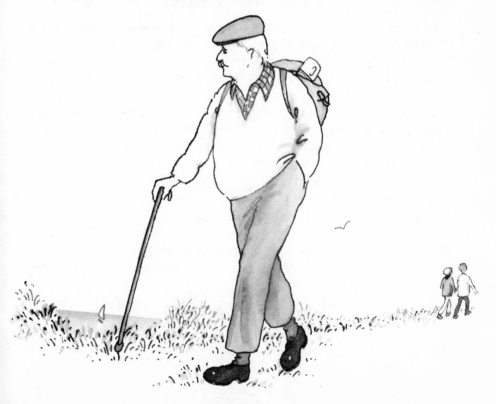

with better times than many in the younger groups. The track walk was split up in groups and competing in the race for competitors of 65+, he finished second overall, winning the 75–79 title in 29 minutes 24.4 seconds. Third overall in the championship was his old friend Gus, now 80, and winner of his group with a time of 30 minutes 42 seconds. (The 20-kilometers included Sweden's extraordinary 84-year-old Fritz Schreiber, still going strong.)

"As you see," Bob concluded, "I overcame many physical handicaps by walking myself to fitness. I have even come to see the setbacks as beneficial. They call a compulsory halt to activity and allow me to recharge my batteries. Incidentally, I have just won a 5-mile race in 48 minutes 38 seconds, a world record for my age. Now I'm looking forward to the 1979 championships in Hanover, Germany. To anyone who thinks of giving up because of age, I say this: whatever the trouble, persevere. A return to health and strength is reward enough: and achievement offers a marvelous additional sense of satisfaction."

Heart-Attack Patients: A Second Chance for Life

Until about twenty years ago, a heart attack was, to all intents and purposes, the end of an active life. Any additional strain on a damaged heart was considered potentially fatal and heart-attack victims were told that their heart had issued its own warning: Don't strain me or else. "Be careful," heart patients were told. "Don't climb stairs too quickly; don't run; give up tennis; resign from the golf club." Tens of thousands of people who were quite capable of living a normal life after a period of recuperation were condemned to what now seems like little more than a living death.

Fortunately, it is now recognized that this is simply not necessary. Just the opposite. A damaged heart, can, in the vast majority of cases, be strengthened again sufficiently not only to take on the burdens of life the victims had been handling up until their attack, but much more – to effect what can literally seem like a rejuvenation.

One way to recovery is by eating well. The clinical benefits of a healthy diet have been researched at the Universities of

Iowa and Chicago in work on monkeys. The monkeys were first given a diet high in saturated fat and cholesterol, and their arteries duly became narrower. They became potential heart-attack victims. Then the monkeys were returned to what the researchers called a "prudent" low-fat diet. Their arteries widened again and their health virtually returned to normal.

The evidence as it applies to human beings is rather more complex because of the many other elements in the diet which are hard to identify. But there are other suggestive pieces of evidence. In Europe, during the Second World War, when there was a general shortage of meat, eggs and animal fats, every European country noted a decrease in fatalities from heart disease – except Denmark: the Danes, traditional exporters of dairy produce, went on eating as before.

The dietary evidence has been sufficient for the Royal College of Physicians in London to recommend a post-heart-attack diet as an aid to recovery:

1. Restrict meat meals to eight a week.
2. Always use soft margarines high in polyunsaturates.
3. Use skimmed milk.
4. Eat no more than three eggs a week.
5. Cut down on cheeses – use cottage cheese whenever possible.
6. Restrict your intake of cakes, pastries, etc., unless made with polyunsaturates.

A vegetarian diet also seems to be particularly effective. The Seventh Day Adventists, whose diet is very strongly vegetarian, have a much lower incidence of heart disease then the population at large (they smoke less and drink less as well, which may also contribute to their good health). It should be emphasized that, although a vegetarian diet may be healthier in our industrialized urban world than one consisting largely of marbled steak, eggs, cheese and fried foods, no diet has been shown to have the miraculous properties that its more way-out adherents claim for it.

But diet is only one element – and a controversial one – in recuperating from a heart attack. The really revolutionary factor – one that means a new life for anyone who survives a heart attack – is walking. And that need only be a beginning. Once bitten by the fitness bug, many heart-attack patients go on to do more strenuous sports than they would ever have imagined possible in middle age. Heart-attack patients now regularly run in the Boston Marathon every year, and they're all the better for it.

The benefits of exercise to a heart-attack patient were described to me by Ian Anderson. "The other day, a 52-year-old man came to see me. He was a company director, well-established. He had had a coronary. It had been pretty severe and he'd been told by his consultant that he could never climb stairs again. Now, that's really harsh. It revealed an attitude in the medical profession that I thought must be almost extinct. Anyway, he told me when he arrived that he could never come to see me again because my offices were up one flight of stairs. That was six weeks after his coronary. Well, we put him on the treadmill and set him walking at two miles an hour. He wasn't in such bad shape as he thought. He came back three times a week and we put him through a carefully monitored program on the treadmill. He could equally well have done it for himself outside, though I would have made sure he took it at a slower pace. That was a year ago. Now he's been posted to New York.

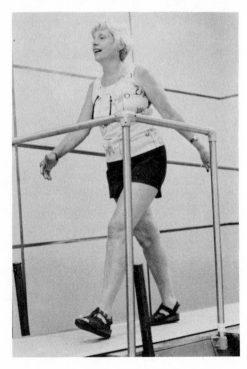

Heart attack victims (here and opposite) walking their way back to health in the controlled, yet relaxed environment of a cardiac rehabilitation center.

He wrote to me the other day. He says he's progressed from walking to occasional jogging. He plays softball and basketball, and he's never felt fitter.

"We've had countless cases like this: heart-attack patients who come in, go through a physical fitness program for a few weeks and are then reassessed. The external conditions are the same at the beginning and end of the program. Always, without exception, there's an improvement – the heart's stronger, and can take more strain; the rhythm has improved; and suddenly the people who came to me as patients are not patients anymore. They are perfectly fit individuals, capable of living their own lives without medical supervision, and perhaps fitter than they've ever been in the last twenty years.

"From a major cardiac event, you can get people fit in ten weeks. The only physical constraint we put on them is to ask them not to play competitive sports like squash or badminton. Now, ten weeks is fairly intensive, but on a treadmill and with an EKG (ECG), you can monitor the heart's reactions by the split second. You can't do that for everyone. Outside the program is slower, but it's equally effective."

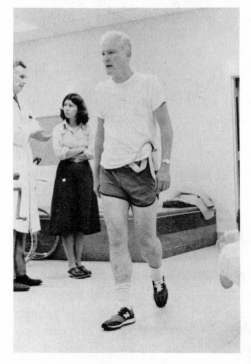

This patient is wearing a telemetry unit that monitors his heart automatically.

129

What are the risks of taking exercise after a heart attack? There is now a huge body of evidence from which to draw some conclusions. There are some half-million post-heart-attack patients in the United States alone. Thousands have been rehabilitated through an exercise program. In supervised programs there is a US national average of one life-threatening event for approximately 30,000 man hours, reports Mike Pollack. It is, therefore, a reassuringly safe activity.

In another study done at the Institute of Physiological Hygiene in Tel-Aviv on 101 coronary patients two years after their attack, the dangers of postcoronary exercise was measured. The patients were divided into two groups. One group was put through a rehabilitation exercise program. The second group took no exercise. At the end of the year, only 10 percent of the nonexercisers said they were free from all angina pectoris pains and over a third of them complained of severe anginal pains. Among the exercisers, however, over 33 percent said they were completely free from anginal pains and only 6 percent complained of severe pains.

The return to an active life must begin under medical supervision, but once out and about – with the occasional checkup – the results can be dramatic. A standard prescription might consist of light calisthenics for warm-up and flexibility; ten minutes of brisk walking, which might take the pulse up to 120 beats per minute; some more rapid walking if the heart can take it; and a final five minutes of warm-down – similar to the plan outlined in Appendices 3 and 4 of "The Walker's Yellow Pages." The effects, too, are comparable. To quote one medical paper by Dr. Arthur Leon, associate professor of medicine at the University of Minnesota: "Adaptive cardiovascular changes . . . resemble those occurring in healthy sedentary people who enter exercise conditioning programs." The heart rate goes down, the blood pressure goes down, blood flow increases.

But perhaps more significant are the wider ranging changes in life style that often occur after a heart attack. The heart-attack patient has had direct contact with doctors in a unique and shocking way and will often come away from the experience with a detailed knowledge of his own body and of what brought on the heart attack. From then on, he and the doctor cooperate in ensuring that he stays out of medical hands from then on. Typically, he'll cut down on, or give up, cigarette smoking and he will lose weight. As his health improves, he will begin to sleep better. Above all, the exercise program will help him to overcome the almost inevitable depression that follows a heart attack. This single factor can be as debilitating for the post-heart-attack patient as his physical disabilities.

One of the most depressing facts about having had a heart attack is that for a few weeks the patient cannot risk indulging in any violent activity, even if it's for a very short period. Now there is one male activity associated with a healthy life that is forbidden to a patient soon after his attack: sex. A recent study of the demands of sexual intercourse on post-heart-attack victims done by Dr. Lenore Zohman, director of Cardiopulmonary Rehabilitation at Montefiore Hospital and Medical Center in New York City, showed that peak heart rates ranged between 101 and 121 beats per minute. The average was 117. For somebody with a damaged heart, this is quite a strain. The strain is intense enough with long-time marital partners (it was from married couples that Dr. Zohman drew their peak heart rate figures). Although there are no figures to support the generali-

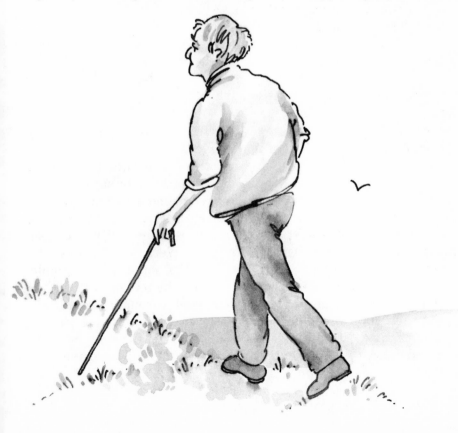

zation, it is known that more men with heart disease have an attack while having an extramarital affair. It is, apparently, more physically demanding and certainly more stressful. These findings have inspired a certain amount of ribald comment in the medical profession, hence the following verses "On Coronary Coupling":

> Coronary, have a care,
> Think before that new affair;
> Dr. Zohman studied swingers
> And her facts are really zingers.
>
> Sex domestic, also straight,
> Hardly makes you palpitate;
> Heart beats stay at normal rate
> When one beds with legal mate,
> And the danger that it bears
> Looms like – well, two sets of stairs.
>
> But roosting in another's nest
> Flirts with cardiac arrest;
> End result of evening's sport is
> Very often rigor mortis.
> So seduction's needs are three –
> Soft lights, music, EKG.

Simple abstinence is not, of course, the answer. This merely accentuates the feelings of inadequacy. What the patient needs is a return to normal – and the quickest way to return to normal is to get out there and walk as soon as your doctor says you can.

Almost all of us have come across someone who can now look forward positively to a healthy old age as a result of their brush with death. And almost everyone shares a similarity of experience. Let the case of Arthur Gordon, a West Coast representative for the publisher Grosset and Dunlap, serve as an example. "It happened a year ago, when I was 64," he told me. "I had had the usual examinations and even went through stress tests, but there didn't seem to be anything wrong with me. Then one day at home, I felt faint, with a constriction over my heart. It was over in a few moments, but I was taken into intensive care. It gave me quite a shock, I can tell you."

"The doctor put me on a gradual program. At first I was walking two blocks very slowly, but I put up my speed and distance a little bit every week. After four months, I was walking for 1½ miles twice a day and after six months, about three miles at the rate of fifteen minutes a mile. That's 4 MPH, and now the doctor doesn't want to see me for a year."

"Diet? That hasn't been so important for me. I didn't have to modify my diet very much. I cut down on cholesterol a bit, but I attribute most of my recovery to walking."

Walking is now part of Arthur Gordon's life. It's not only a physical, but an emotional rebirth. "I like it best early in the morning, before the traffic, when the air's fresh. That's when it helps my mental state best. It's a time of introspection and relaxation for me."

Several thousands of patients have now had the benefits of a careful analysis of their exercise needs and a long-term training program.

Dr. Kattus, chairman of the Exercise Committee of the American Heart Association, and professor of medicine at the University of California, Los Angeles, described his own program. "My walking patients are unsupervised, mainly because it's difficult in California to get people to come together in a gym. They're disseminated over a wide area and the weather is suitable for them to do outdoor exercise on their own, so we have tailored our program accordingly. Even if the patients have significant heart disease, we simply have to assay the level of hazard and instruct them so that they'll stay below that." Sometimes patients are monitored by telemetry. They're always instructed about how to take their own pulse.

The result is that all across North America and increasingly throughout the United Kingdom and elsewhere, heart patients are recovering secure in the knowledge that they're being looked after and can eventually look after themselves, confident in their growing physical capacity and also reinforced by contact with others in the same situation.

Finally, it's worth a reminder that once heart patients are up and about again, they can be regarded as a normal beginner in the basic walking program. They can slot themselves straight into their own fitness level, according to "The Walker's Yellow Pages." Soon they will no longer be patients. They will be walkers, and fitter than they've ever been before.

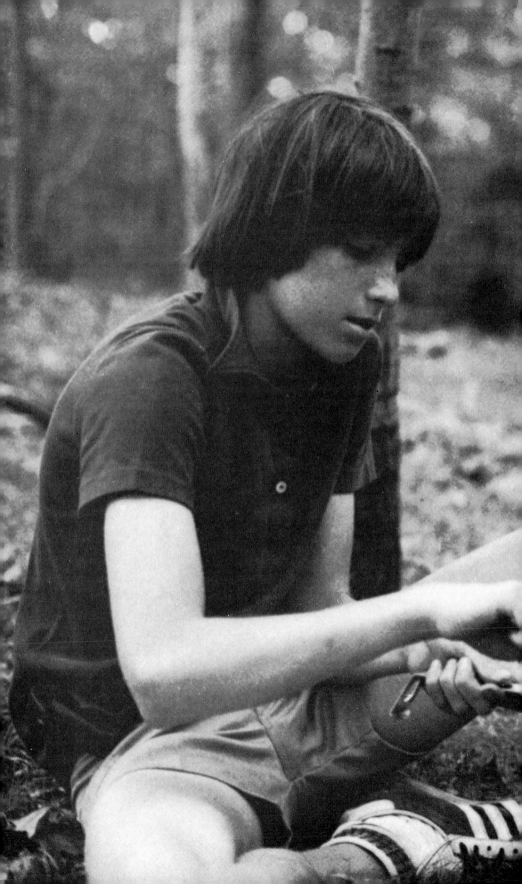

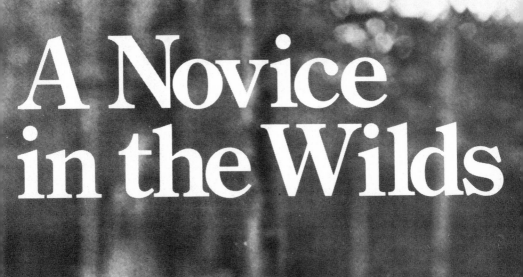

A Novice
in the Wilds

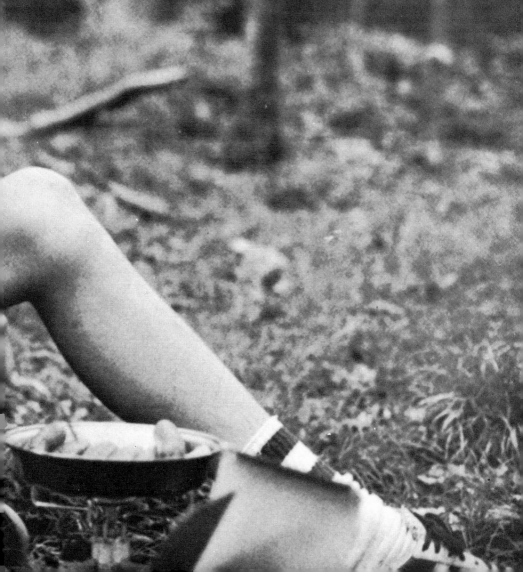

A Novice in the Wilds

I WANT TO TALK FOR a moment or two about the joys and tribulations of backpacking. The English don't make much of a formal distinction between those who simply head into the country for a day's walk and those who set off for weeks at a time with "houses" on their back. The Americans, used to greater distances and remoter landscapes, do, and rightly so. Short and long-distance walking may not differ much in terms of the quality of the experience, but in terms of planning and energy expenditure they certainly do.

I am not a backpacker of many years' standing. I'm a newcomer; and since I am probably talking to newcomers, I would like to think this is a qualification. Trained backpackers take a lot for granted. They devote much expert attention to the planning of routes; they debate the finer points of specialized equipment; but the actual business of carrying a pack has become overfamiliar. If you want the flavor of a first-time experience, stay with me.

First, a word of warning: carrying a pack is surprisingly demanding. I was vacationing with my children recently near Salcombe in South Devon. We were at a beach. Sloping up from it was a grassy hillside leading to a craggy cliff-top path. It climbed steeply at an angle of perhaps 30 degrees for about 120 yards to a crest 100 feet above the sea. I decided to do an experiment to see just how demanding carrying a heavy pack can be. I had no pack, but thought that my six-year-old daughter, Emily, who tips the scales at 50 pounds, would do as a substitute.

"Come on," I called to her, "I'm going to carry you up the hill." As we both get older, and she gets heavier, that's not the sort of offer that comes her way often. As she ran over, I took

---

"The best preparation for a walking holiday lies not in fine weather so much as in hard feet, and to get the feet hard there is but one way, and that is by walking."

A. N. Cooper, *A Holiday on Tramp*

---

my resting heart beat; it was 60. I jumped her up on my shouldders and set off. It took me 2½ minutes to reach the top. Slow going, you may think; but when I arrived at the crest, I was thoroughly spent. My heart rate had risen to 140, but this did not really reflect the exhaustion I felt. My calf and thigh muscles were screaming, and the small of my back ached.

The conclusion is clear-cut: physically, walking with a pack is superb exercise, once you're fit enough to take it. If you did a climb equivalent to mine a few times a week, you would be doing enough to keep heart and muscles in better-than-average shape.

I won't go very deeply into the technical details of backpacking, because there are numerous publications and books (some of them mentioned in the Bibliography), whose authors are far better qualified than I am to offer such advice. All I can do is provide a brief summary of some of the most basic things you should be aware of. Then, for those who want to give it a try (and also for those who want to relive their first tentative steps with pack on back) I will describe what I imagine is a fairly typical first-time experience – a brief, tiring, but exhilarating walk on the Appalachian Trail in New York State.

Training

If you are out of trim or have never carried a pack before, it will take you anything up to three months to get to the point where you can carry a 30- or 40-pound load easily and comfortably for several days. It takes time to accommodate to the feel of the thing. It alters your balance. You have to lean forward and your arms tend to droop until you feel like a caricature of a Neanderthal man. You tend to walk flatfootedly. Hips and shoulders ache easily. You feel unaccustomed pressure in your knees. A friend of mine once headed for the Welsh hills with visions of covering many miles a day for two weeks. After one day, he took a train back, incapacitated by soreness and swearing never to carry a pack again.

It is the hills that really get to you. You tend to climb with your toes, and you will find that, after a few hundred paces of climbing with a pack on your back, your calves will not be able to take the strain. Even experienced walkers need to get back into trim. Both Colin Fletcher, whose witty and practical *The Complete Walker* is the American backpacker's bible, and John Hillaby, well-known in England for his writings on long-distance walking, advise strapping weights into a pack and getting out and about for several weeks before the start of the trip to harden up the body. As Colin Fletcher says, "You may blench at the thought of pounding up Main Street with a 40-pound pack, but pray, what are city parks for?" Because going uphill is about ten times harder than walking on the flat, there is really no alternative for the would-be backpacker who wants to get in trim but to – you've guessed it – walk uphill with a pack.

Equipment

Packs

The pack is, of course, the core of the matter. Packs, as they have evolved over the last fifteen years or so, have revolutionized the sport. Firstly, they are now light with strong aluminum frames and synthetic fiber containers. And secondly almost all of them have waistbelts, which must rank as one of this century's truly great inventions.

One thing that surprised me when I recently took to the trail with a pack was the amount my hips ached. The only previous time I had carried a pack, which was about twenty years ago, my shoulders almost gave way. The only thing supporting the weight of the pack was its shoulder straps. Nowadays most packs have waistbelts which transfer much of the weight to the top of the legs. This is a far more efficient way of dealing with weight than having it all hanging off the top of your spine. It does, however, put an unaccustomed strain on the hips and they will protest. But stay with it: they adapt.

There are three main things I think should be stressed about a waistbelt: it should be wide; it should be padded; and it should completely encircle you. This last point is particularly

The Bad Old Days – I

Backpacking inspires considerable enjoyment but little wit among its adherents. Pat McManus is an exception: his is a voice laughing in the wilderness. His monthly contributions to Field and Stream *have for years recorded the comic side of living in the wild. This extract and the one on page 158 are taken from his book* A Fine and Pleasant Misery *(New York: Holt, Rinehart and Winston).*

The rule of thumb for the old backpacking was that the weight of your pack should equal the weight of yourself and the kitchen range combined. Just a casual glance at a full pack sitting on the floor could give you a double hernia and fuse four vertebrae. After carrying the pack all day, you had to remember to tie one leg to a tree before you dropped it. Otherwise, you would float off into space. The pack eliminated the need for any special kind of ground-gripping shoes, because your feet would sink a foot and a half into hard-packed earth, two inches into solid rock. Some of the new breed of backpackers occasionally wonder what caused a swath of fallen trees on the side of a mountain. That is where one of the old backpackers slipped off a trail with a full pack.

My packboard alone met the minimum weight requirement. It was a canvas and plywood model, surplus from the Second World War. These packboards apparently were designed with the idea that a number of them could be hooked together to make an emergency bridge for Sherman tanks . . .

My sleeping bag looked like a rolled-up mattress salvaged from a fire in a skid row hotel. Its filling was sawdust, horsehair, and No. 6 bird shot. Some of today's backpackers tell me their sleeping bags are so light they scarcely know they're there. The only time I scarcely knew my sleeping bag was there was when I was in it at 2 a.m. on a cold night. It was freckled from one end to the other with spark holes, a result of my efforts to stay close enough to the fire to keep warm. The only time I was halfway comfortable was when it was ablaze. It was the only sleeping bag I ever heard of which you could climb into in the evening with scarcely a mark on you and wake up in the morning bruised from head to toe. That was because two or three times a night my companions would take it upon themselves to jump up and stomp out my sleeping-bag fires – in their haste neglecting to first evacuate the occupant. Since I was the camp cook, I never knew whether they were attempting to save me from immolation or getting in a few last licks for what they thought might be terminal indigestion.

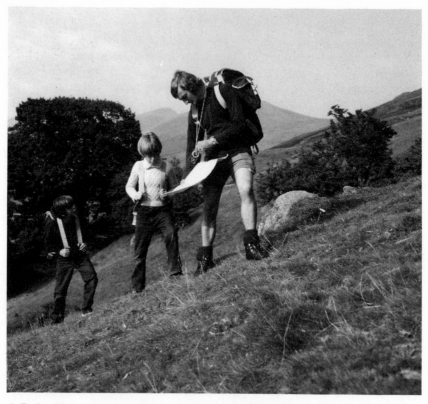

A Lake District rambler and his two children examine a map.

important. If you are tempted, for the sake of the price, to go for a pack with a belt that consists of side straps attached directly to the base of the frame, *don't* be; the band will take little weight from the shoulders and the sides of the frame can rub you sore in no time. Physically and psychologically, a waistbelt takes the weight off your shoulders. When you first sling a pack on your back, the weight seems formidable, but as soon as you hitch the waistbelt into position and haul it onto a tight notch – it should always be worn tight – the weight seems to drop away to nothing.

The only other thing that seems vital to me is that the shoulder straps should also be padded. You cannot expect to get the full emotional and physical benefit from walking if your equipment is uncomfortable.

To the uninitiated, packs look like nothing more than piles of odd sacking. In fact, there is a wealth of thinking behind the

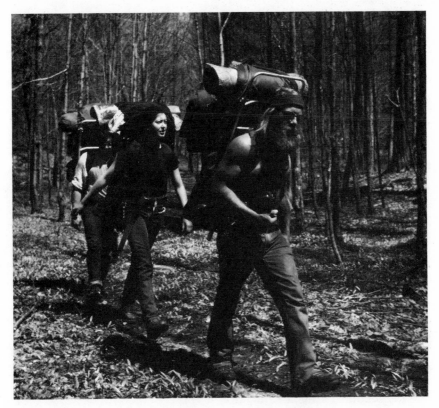

The American way: hanging loose on the Hippie Trail.

design. Once you get into the subject you risk being baffled by
the range and positioning of pockets, flaps, straps, zippers and
ties. Combine this with the different levels of waterproofing
available and the different weights of material and you'll begin
to see the scope of the problem. The only answer is to shortcut
experience by seeking expert guidance.

There is one thing I have promised myself to experiment with
the next time I go backpacking: a chest harness. The purpose of
the shoulder straps is not to carry weight – most of that is
borne by the waistbelt – but to stop the pack falling over backward. I find, at least for me, that there is still some strain,
however, on the shoulders, for the harness tends to slip outward
(hence the habit many backpackers develop of slipping their
thumbs under the straps as they walk). It should be possible to
tie the straps together in front of you so that the remaining
strain is taken more by the chest than the shoulders. Perhaps

some manufacturer somewhere makes an adjustable strap for such a purpose, but so far I haven't heard of one.

Tents

My delight in modern equipment applies equally to tents. Now, there are an infinite variety of tents for every type of environment, season, climate and weather, and for any number of people from a single occupant up to a mini-commune. Some tents are better for wind, others for snow. There are special mountain tents. There are those you can cook in and those you can't. Some have extra flaps to form an additional storage area outside the tent. Some have foul-weather sleeves to get in by. If you want to live really simply, you can even rig up a variety of shelters with a ground sheet and a bit of string slung between two trees.

Again, if you want details, it is best to analyze your needs and consult a good dealer. But there are a few personal things I'd like to say about tents. For my choice, they should be all-in-one, with ground-sheet attached and without any gaps in the seams. If there are gaps, "things" (like rain and ants, for starters) will get in. Whatever they are, I would always rather they were out.

The second thing a tent should have is mosquito netting on the inside of all windows, fine enough to keep out all known forms of insect. I find that zippers, too, are essential – no tie-up flaps for me. Modern zippers are bug-proof, almost waterproof, do not rust and are quick to use. Finally, if you really want your money's worth, I suggest you consider a tent that does not have center poles. There are many tents available with supports that consist of rods which, when set up, bend to fit the various edges of the tent and keep it in shape by pressure alone. This arrangement not only ensures that the synthetic skin remains pleasingly taut, but makes much more room inside.

One other point on tents: ask yourself if you really need one. I have slept out only once, a long time ago, when I was about 15. I was in an orchard, near my home in Kent, and remember looking up past the apple branches at the velvet, star-pointed sky. The oddly secure feeling of being part of the canopy of the universe has stayed with me ever since.

I was reminded of this when I recently came across this passage by Colin Fletcher:

Some worlds only come alive after dark, and my memory often cheers me with little cameos it would not hold if I always roofed myself off from the night. Deep in Grand Canyon, inches from my eyes, floodlit by flashlight, a pair of quick, clean little deer mice scamper with thistledown delicacy along slender willow shoots. On a Cornish hillside, with the Atlantic pounding away at the cliffs below, the shadowy shape of a fox ambles unconcernedly out and then back into the darkness. . . . Without a roof, you wake directly into the new day. Sometimes I open my eyes in the morning to see a rabbit bobbing and nibbling its way through breakfeast. Once I woke at dawn to find, ten feet from my head, a doe browsing among dew-covered ferns.

Boots and Other Protective Gear

There is a good deal of conflicting information and evidence here. The advantages of boots are obvious: they keep out the wet (if properly treated); they protect the soles from stones; and they offer support for the ankles. The Ramblers' Association in London is explicit enough in their recommendation: "Specialized walking boots are essential for comfort and confidence if you aim to walk all the year round and over any mountainous and moorland country." But note the qualification: *if* you walk the year round and *if* you walk in mountains and moorlands.

The other side of this argument is that if you are not a confirmed long-distance, all-weather, rough-country walker, you can save yourself money (boots cost a small fortune) and trouble (they also take time to wear in). John Hillaby, who has many thousands of miles beneath his soles, despises traditional hiker's boots. "I know of nothing more uncomfortable," he says. "They give you a leaden, nonspringy stride. You can't trot along in boots." He prefers a light-weight pair. I like heavy-duty sneakers for summer use (I don't mind wet feet as long as it's warm), but use boots, of course, for winter and rough-country work.

You will also need protection against rain (walking in the rain is a pleasure all on its own but if you're on a long walk, you probably won't want to get your clothing wet). There is the usual baffling range to choose from. Avoid "showerproof" garments. They often look nice, but if you took the manufacturers at their word and stepped under a shower in one you would be soaked through in no time. Assume it will rain, and rain hard, and that you will be caught in the downpour. Buy a totally waterproof covering: the material is light and easy to pack away. It does tend to "sweat" with condensation but I haven't found this much of an inconvenience.

To keep the knees dry, walking manuals usually advise sack-like things called cagoules, which come way down over the knees. In principle, these are fine, but they never seem to keep the legs quite as dry as they should. The next time I go any distance, I'll take along waterproof trousers as a match for the jacket I wear, which is zippered. (The pull-over varieties demand ungainly calisthenics to get on and off; and with a zipper you can air yourself out if you get too hot.)

There is one thing I find enormously useful, which not many jackets provide: a peaked hood. Your average, run-of-the-mill hood has a string which you tie up underneath your chin. I find this kind of hood has two disadvantages: it tends to drift around your head and blocks your vision; and it does nothing to shelter your face from the rain. Hoods with peaks don't slide around, and can guarantee a drier-eyed view of the world.

Walking Softly

Let's now assume you have perused your catalogs, taken the advice of your local outdoor sports stores, bought what you need and that you are ready to head off into the wilds. Though you may think you are heading for solitude, you are only partially right. You will be joining a veritable army of back-packers and ramblers who annually invade the wilds of America and Europe. Hiking is a fast-growing pastime. In 1950 Americans spent about four million twelve-hour days hiking with packs. In 1978 the figure was fifty million. Wilderness hiking has grown about five times as fast as the population.

The result of this invasion has been, predictably, crisis – especially in the United States, where so many people now seek the joys of wilderness travel that they risk destroying the very benefits they seek. Given the vast areas they have at their disposal, this may seem startling. America's Wilderness Preservation System, established by the Wilderness Act of 1964, incorporates some 127 areas – about thirteen million acres in all. Legislation now pending could, if passed, triple this amount. This sounds adequate to accommodate any amount of hikers

"Going tramping is at first an act of rebellion; only afterwards do you get free from rebelliousness as Nature sweetens your mind. Town makes men contentious; the country smooths out their souls."

Stephen Graham, *The Gentle Art of Tramping*

(though it is in fact just 1.6 percent of the total area of the US), but it must be remembered that some places are more heavily used than others. There is, to use the current jargon, an "impact problem." Around popular campsites, woods have been stripped of young growth by walkers hunting for fuel. Meadows have been flattened. Fire is a constant hazard. Popular trails are littered with paper bags, bottles and discarded food, constant reminders of the presence of others.

The individual walker seeking solitude – and that is what most of us do seek – can and should be prepared to minimize the problems. In areas where unrestricted camping is allowed (and some argue that this makes better sense than polluting acres with vast campsites), there are certain rules that every walker should adopt. Together these form a style of backpacking termed "going light" by John Hart, in the Sierra Club's superb guide to backpacking *Walking Softly in the Wilderness*. In summary, "going light" means:

Never light a fire. Take a stove with you. Although fires are a traditional part of the camping ritual, they may destroy the fertility of the soil, leave scars on rocks, consume green wood and burn away dry meadowland. There are, of course, many places where a fire is safe – in open woodlands well supplied with fallen branches and with a stony soil, for instance – but it is still better not to be tempted.

Don't camp on meadowland or at the edge of a wood. Grasses and new growth are easily destroyed. Better to camp in the wood itself.

Choose a sight where you do not have to dig ditches, pile up stones or cut down branches. It is better to preserve than to pioneer.

Carry your trash with you. Nothing is more revolting to new arrivals than the rotting evidence of previous inhabitants. (I was once walking around Loch Ness, in Scotland. It was late September. The Loch was beautifully ominous, still and brooding. Yet the mood was spoiled at every turn of the footpath not only by the patches of flattened grass and fire scars, but by Coke cans, candy wrappers, plastic bags, string, cardboard boxes and other eyesores. No wonder Nessie keeps to the depths.)

Which Way? . . . and Right of Way

Bearing all this in mind, you're ready to set off.

But where? You can, of course, walk almost anywhere, as long as you do not infringe on private property. In fact, the easiest form of hiking is to choose an established route. It is easier to plan and safer: and you can travel further and faster. In terms of exercise, you get a better return from time invested. Any national park has miles of trails to be followed. Or you can venture onto the long-distance paths like England's Pennine Way or the Appalachian Trail, which stretches for two thousand miles from Maine to Georgia.

The Appalachian Trail was first suggested in 1921 in the *Journal of the American Institute of Architects* by forester and author Benton Mackaye. In 1925 a number of local wilderness groups joined together and formed the Appalachian Trail Conference to coordinate the clearing and marking of the trail. Today it is the longest marked path in the world and justifiably the most famous.

Throughout most of its length the Appalachian Trail fulfills its original purpose: to provide access to primeval natural environments for anyone who wishes to walk in them. But the balance between retaining the primeval quality of the wilderness and supplying the needs of wilderness travelers is a precarious one that needs continual monitoring. One of the policies of the Trail Conference, for instance, has been to provide lean-to shelters for campers. This philanthropic gesture has led to problems, as I learned from George Zoebelein, who for many years was a prime mover in the Trail Conference. "The shelters attract day trippers who have no intention of walking the trail," he explained. "They park their cars at the nearest road, stroll into the woods and set up house for days at a time. When the shelters are not used, they're often vandalized. When they are used, they are often overcrowded, and tend to form a scar on the wilderness. Financially and ecologically, I don't think we can afford them." He hinted that the trail users will be left to rely more on their own resources, camping where they wish.

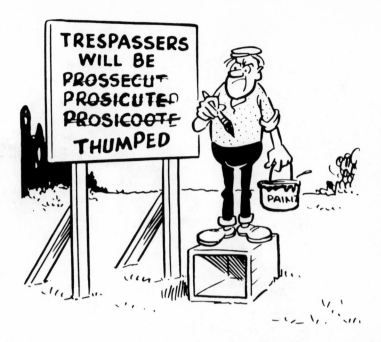

This should be good news for walkers. As long as they recognize their responsibilities toward the trail and to others who use it, it will perhaps fulfill its original purpose even better in the future than it has in the past.

In England the 30,000-strong Rambler's Association, based in London, has numerous local groups whose members between them share the task of organizing walks between five and twenty miles long through the local countryside. There's no easier way to get to know the trails than by going along with someone who can show you the way. If you enjoy meeting (and walking with) new people with similar interests, then rambling might be just your cup of tea.

Wherever you walk, though, unless you stick to the major marked trails, you must face the problem of access. All land nowadays is owned by somebody, even if it is the state, and in Britain, walkers – in the form of the Rambler's Association and the Commons and Footpath Preservation Society – fight a continuous battle about rights of access. Traditionally, access is sanctioned only by acknowledged historic right, and this is extremely hard to establish. To determine the status of a footpath – when a landowner, for instance, wanted to close a

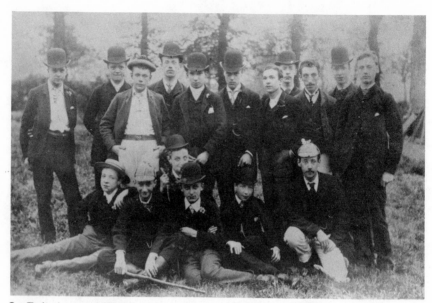

In Britain rambling is a long-established pastime. Here, formally attired for the camera, are the members of London's Polytechnic Rambling Club of 1885.

particular way – it was once necessary to establish legally that the path had in fact been used for so long as to justify the assumption that a former owner had once sanctioned the right of access. Since 1949, however, when the National Parks and Access to the Countryside Act was passed, county councils have been drawing up a definitive map showing all rights of way, legally secured (until, that is, they come up for review). If you leave the established path, you may technically be committing a trespass. But you can be prosecuted only in a civil action and only to the extent of the damage you cause: so the signs "TRESPASSERS WILL BE PROSECUTED," still common in the English countryside, are practically meaningless unless you have the unpleasant experience of coming up against a surly and resentful landowner.

In Britain you can roam freely in those areas covered by access agreements or orders made by local authorities under the 1949 National Parks Act. There is, in addition, a mass of other pockets of land, known as commons, where local people, or commoners, were traditionally allowed to graze cattle or gather wood or peat for fuel, but there was never a general public right of access to commons. The Commons Society

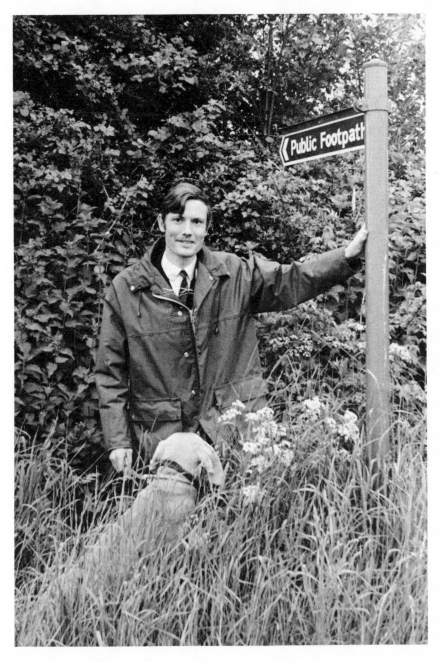

A man and his dog in search of a footpath—an age-old problem in Britain. Public footpaths, though sanctioned by centuries of use, are often overgrown or closed. Ramblers fight tenaciously to keep them open.

149

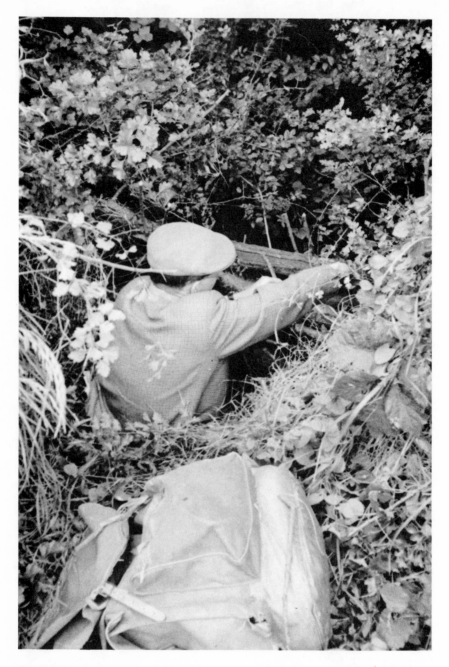

The problems of access: a rambler in the English countryside near Uffington, Berkshire, with a gate barring a path to which access is legally guaranteed by centuries of use—as long as that right is exercised.

estimates that some 360,000 acres (about a quarter of the total commons areas) are open to the public; but this is by custom, not by right. In addition, the Forestry Commission and the National Trust generally allow public access.

Legal battles over the status of footpaths can go on for many years, as exemplified by the case of Wychwood Forest, some twenty miles north of Oxford. Wychwood was a royal forest that once covered a great stretch of west Oxfordshire. Right up to the mid-nineteenth century, travelers freely made their way through. Then in 1857 it was closed by a deforestation award that led to the felling of vast areas of the forest and its partial conversion into arable land. The remnant – present-day Wychwood Forest – lay in a little populated area and few footpaths were established. In 1949 the chairman of the local organization, whose task it was to draw the footpaths, was the owner. He was careful not to include paths across his own property. Local villagers and interested councillors protested; appeals were lodged to reinstate just one path; enquiries were held; but despite the centuries of use, there was a vital gap in the late nineteenth century, and it is impossible now to bring forward witnesses who could testify to the regular use of the path in question. One up to the owners (although every Palm Sunday, by ancient custom, a path in the forest of Wychwood is briefly open to the public, at which time the place is alive with visitors asserting their historic right; if the path were ever opened again, there could be no risk of its falling into disuse a second time).

In the US the problem is rather more clear cut and perhaps a little less urgent because of the wealth of areas open to the public. Private property is private property and access has to be agreed between state or national authorities and the landowners. The property interest remains the dominant one and the rights can be revoked at any time.

Fear and Loathing on the Appalachian Trail

In June 1978, as I was preparing to make my first trip along the Appalachian Trail, two friends, Desmond Heath, an English psychiatrist who has been living in Manhattan for the last twenty years, and his 14-year-old son Julian, volunteered to

join me. This was something of a windfall. I had little equipment of my own, but the whole Heath family, Desmond, his
wife Susan and their four boys, ranging from 18 to 11, are all
outdoors people. As well as being dedicated city dwellers, they
have an old clapboard farmhouse near Staatsburg, about eighty
miles north of the city, in which they harbored an ill-assorted
collection of frame packs, tents, picnic canteens, parkas and
boots. We would surely be able to put together enough hiking
gear for the three of us.

The greatest attraction of all, however, was a newly acquired
light-weight tent that could sleep six. It was a revelation. I
hadn't examined a tent since I was a teenager, when tents were
heavy and leaked as soon as you touched them. It always
took an hour of hammering pegs and tying guy ropes to get
them up, and they had put me off camping for twenty years.
This new tent, by comparison, was a masterpiece of design, with
four corner posts and a ridge pole which, when slotted together
in a self-stressing arrangement, kept taut the inner skin of the
tent, along with its ground sheet. Outside, a waterproof over-
sheet completed the structure. It weighed just seventeen pounds.
We tried it out in the garden. It took a mere ten minutes to
set up.

The rest of the preparations took rather longer. We made
lists of things that we needed. I bought some basic medical
supplies – Bandaid, corn pads to protect blisters, antiseptic
cream, mosquito repellant (*especially* mosquito repellant). I
wondered whether I would need long trousers or a sweater. But
it was hot, and didn't look like rain. Following Colin Fletcher's
advice, I decided to keep the weight down as much as possible,
and opted to go in shorts, a shirt, socks and my heavy-duty
sneakers, with their thick soles and wrap-around heels. We
packed anoraks, swimming trunks, towels, toothbrushes and
toothpaste. We added knives, forks, spoons, plates, dried soup,
raisins, cereal, sausages, bacon, a canteen of water and even a
small jam jar full of bourbon. All this, together with tent and
sleeping bags, made a considerable bulk. Desmond and I carried
about thirty pounds each, while Julian hefted a lighter load, as
befitted his age and weight.

I had studied the map of the trail for this region and decided
that in the two days that we had at our disposal we should
easily be able to walk down from Canopus Lake, fifteen miles

to Bear Mountain Bridge. After all, I had talked to walkers who could quite happily manage twenty-five miles a day. The others could turn back if they wanted. I even had visions of going on alone, swinging over the Hudson and the Bear Mountain Bridge and taking a quick hike up Bear Mountain itself for a sweeping view of the river. If other people can do twenty-five miles in one day, I reckoned I could do twenty-five miles in two. I didn't want to attempt anything too ferocious. It was, after all, the first time I had ever been out with a pack and my first time in the American wilds.

In the afternoon Susan drove us, armed with the Appalachian Trail guide, down the Taconic Parkway to Canopus Lake. I kept a diary of the trip to ensure I recalled my impressions:

We are standing in the Fahnestock State Park by Canopus Lake. We must look a little baffled, for at first we don't know where to find the trail. Then, with some embarrassment, we see that just ahead of us is a large noticeboard that pinpoints the beginning of the trail, which tumbles off the edge of the road into the woods. We take it. Almost immediately, we come to a fork and have to stop to check the trail guide for directions. A well-kept track heads off into the forest. To our right, there is another, much smaller path. We see a tree bearing two small white rectangular blazes – the mark of the trail. We clamber

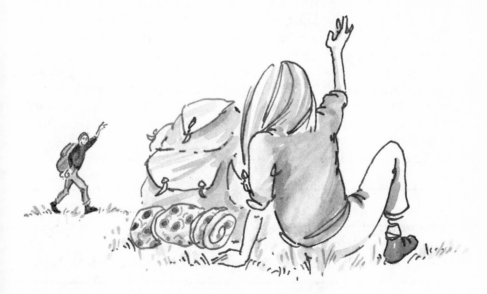

down the eight-foot bank and then set off again. It is a rugged little path, only some eighteen inches wide. It is strewn with boulders from the steep slope along which it winds and is entangled with roots of the surrounding hemlocks. At any one time. I can see a dozen that have fallen downhill, victims of the boulders and top soil that have shifted beneath them over the years.

I see we are halfway up a valley wall that is perhaps two hundred feet from ridge to base. It's five o'clock. The sunlight dapples down through the foliage. Around us all is silent. I see a little note attached to a bush by the side of the trail, placed by an earlier walker, identifying himself (or herself) as "Kluana" from St. Thomas in the Virgin Islands.

As we head into the woodlands, I feel a twinge of nervousness. My socks are well pulled up against poison ivy and I wonder vaguely about the possibility of snakes. At the store this morning when we were buying last-minute provisions, I saw some snake-bite serum. "Do you have snakes in this part of New York?" I asked the assistant. "Oh, yes," she replied cheerfully. But she didn't advise me to buy any.

Nearing the bottom of the valley, we reach a small defile and the trail crosses a little causeway, built up out of local stones. We spot a tree to which is nailed an up-ended box. Inside is a small register book, marked "Appalachian Trail, Maine to Georgia." We put our names in it. Ten other groups have passed here today, thirty-one people all together, an average of only two or three an hour. The trees look a little more stable here, the soil is thicker. There is some grass underfoot. Two chipmunks scamper away in alarm. We move uphill a bit, then on down. I hadn't realized that the backpack would be so noisy. The continual squeak of an eyehole in the waistbelt and the rub of material on material seems to cut me off from the woodlands.

We are heading directly down now, quite steeply, very slowly

"As the day goes on, the traveller . . . becomes more and more incorporated with the material landscape, and the open-air drunkenness grows upon him with great strides."

Robert Louis Stevenson, *Walking Tours*

---

and with considerable effort. With each step, I have to control my momentum. After only a couple of minutes, I can feel the effect in the front of my thighs. We reach the bottom of the valley and make our way past a fetid bog with uprooted trees covered in moss.

We walk the valley floor along a path that wanders between well-spaced trees set in four-inch grass. The land here was once cultivated. There are some ancient apple trees, which must be well over a hundred years old. Desmond remarks: "The ground is so dry it sounds hollow." And indeed, if you stamp, the inches of fallen leaves, built into a felt-like floor over the centuries, gives the same sensation as tapping a dish through cream.

We reach the steep slope at the other side of the valley, and begin to ascend. We slow right down, taking a short pace every second. We stop to rest on a fallen tree, sweating and panting. This is tougher than I thought it would be.

We have been walking for an hour. The guide book says we should emerge very shortly on unpaved road. We breast the top of the hill through a grove of mountain laurel and walk along the crest of a ridge into pine forest. The woodlands are extraordinarily varied. Still and silent enough, perhaps, in our minute-to-minute experience, yet full of change. You can get a good idea of the wood's timetable simply by looking at the fallen trees. After a few minutes, I can make a rough guess at when each of them fell by the state of decay. That one over there, a new casualty; another with peeling bark must have fallen a year ago; a third, which died perhaps five years ago, is already shredded by frost and rain. The track crosses it; and at that point it has been flattened almost beyond recognition.

Now we are going off the ledge in a very steep descent. We climb down, holding onto the roots and rocks. This is definitely not a walk for the unfit. We come to a stream over which three planks are stretched. The stream runs out of an overgrown lake. We decide to take a break. We sit on a rock and look out over the lake. It is in the process of silting up, and dotted across it are the remains of tree trunks. Most likely it is the result of a stream dammed by beavers which has backed up, destroying the trees and creating a whole new ecology.

A few yards offshore somebody is fishing. Behind him towers a boulder, evidence that at least this part of the shore was once dry land. The rest of the lake is clogged with rushes. Perhaps

155

in a century, the rushes will have decayed into mud and the mud provided sustenance for trees. We share a chocolate bar, a sip of water and head off again into the wood.

We come immediately to an unpaved road. A quarter of a mile down a sidetrack, says the guide, there is a small stone structure, complete with spring, that can house ten people. Julian's pack is beginning to bother him a bit. He couldn't get his waistbelt to fit properly and he can't carry more than a few pounds in comfort. It's another mile or so to a paved road where the going will be easier. "Come on," he says, "I can make it." We decide to press on.

For the first time we see evidence that the trail is too often used by inconsiderate walkers – a crumpled cigarette pack that will take a year or so to degrade; a small plastic container blackened with age and sediment, but still as strong as ever; an empty Coke bottle discarded by someone too lazy to carry it out. We, also, are too lazy. I bury it, and feel a pang of conscience, knowing that the next good rain will uncover it again.

We are gradually going uphill. Julian begins to wilt. "Slow down," I say. "Take small steps; just keep going, however slowly. That way, you get into a rhythm." That's what the books say anyway. I hope it's true. I need to get into a rhythm myself. I'm not finding the going easy. We're either climbing with the slope pulling at our calves, or descending with aching thighs. We just have to learn to go slow.

We're quite high now. I catch a glimpse out through the trees of distant forested hills that must be twenty miles away. It makes me wonder how we'd be faring without a trail to follow.

The character of the woods changes again. Scattered stones, lots of dry leaves and twigs, but no other plants except the trees, which are mostly thin, stretching up to the light thirty or forty feet above. Every now and then a mast-like tulip tree, with densely grained, wrinkled bark, drives up from the forest floor, capping its rivals by a good twenty feet.

I've gradually become aware of my ankles. I'm wearing my tough Levi sneakers but now I can see the advantages of wearing really strong hiking boots. The rocks jut out threateningly in places. Roots weave up unexpectedly. If you twisted your ankle, you'd have to be carried out. With the weight of the pack, every slight turn of the ankle makes me think of the dangers of a sprain.

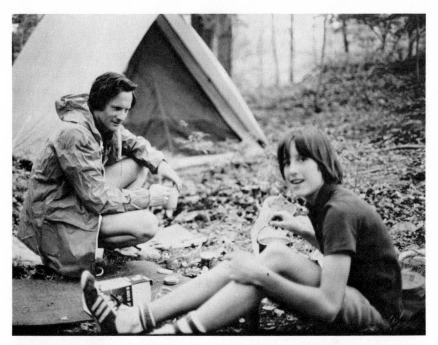

Camping in Fahnestock Park, New York: Julian serves up a simple breakfast.

We emerge onto a second paved road. A sign points us toward a well, a quarter of a mile in the wrong direction. We need to replenish our water. We stroll along until we come to the well, a standpipe in the ground. A child, about seven years old, informs us that there is a campsite nearby. We are debating whether to move toward it, when from the woods there emerges a woman of extraordinary beauty in a long peasant skirt and halter top.

"Is there a campsite here?" I ask her. She gives me a dazzling smile, looks me straight in the eye and says: "Sure, we have a campsite here. You're welcome to join us." We all decide that a campsite could be of more than passing interest. "Yes," she continues, "why *don't* you join us?" But there is something that gives me pause in her generosity. "We are a Christian community from Connecticut. We have fifty-nine children and twenty-seven adults, and we would be glad to have you join our Sunday service tomorrow morning."

I might have known. Nothing to do with my rugged good looks at all. Ah, well.

The Bad Old Days – II

Pat McManus, author of A Fine and Pleasant Misery, *takes a witty look at the horrors of campsite cuisine.*

Our provisions were not distinguished by variety. Dehydrated foods were considered effeminate. A man could ruin his reputation for life by getting caught on a pack trip with a dried apple. If you wanted apples, brother, you carried them with the water still in them. No one could afford such delicacies as commercial beef jerky. What you carried was a huge slab of bacon. It was so big that if the butcher had left on the legs, it could have walked behind you on a leash.

A typical meal consisted of fried bacon, potatoes and onions fried in bacon grease, a pan of beans heated in bacon grease, bacon grease gravy, some bread fried in bacon grease, and cowboy coffee (made by boiling an old cowboy in bacon grease). After meals, indigestion went through our camp like a sow grizzly with a toothache. During the night coyotes sat in nervous silence on surrounding hills and listened to the mournful wailing from our camp.

We stroll up through a plantation of pines to have a look at the camp. There are about twenty-five tents with dozens of children, all busy flattening a meadow. A campfire is blazing in the middle of the circle of tents. It is not the sort of wilderness we're looking for.

Besides, I am keen to camp in the woods. I remember the Sierra Club's advice against camping in fields to prevent any damage to grass. So we back off and find a spot in the woods about half a mile away, clear of undergrowth and soft with fallen leaves. An ideal site.

Desmond sweeps a space clear of twigs and we unload. Julian sets up the stove and begins to lay out a random selection of food – raisins, cereal, sausages. Up goes the tent. We share bourbon from the jam jar. We are, as they say in the children's books, tired but happy. The woodlands are soft around us in the dying light of the day. It is a beautiful experience, and worth a month's walking, let alone a few hours.

I have brought no air mattress. But the leaves are soft. The only thing I miss is an air pillow, which I'll be sure to bring next time.

Up at 6:45. A perfect morning. Utter stillness except for the electric hum of horseflies, which hover as individuals, each, apparently, over its own territory. I stroll around the site, smelling the new day and reveling in the swish of fallen leaves.

Desmond and Julian get up and we take almost an hour over a leisurely breakfast of cinnamon-flavored instant Quaker oatmeal with apples and raisins. Then we set off along a small country road, through woodlands that perhaps a century ago were open farmlands, but are now reverting to true wilderness. It will be a mile or so before we get back into the woods. We crack along at about four miles an hour, at least double what we can manage in the woods.

Julian breaks into song, Jackson Browne's

> *Oh, won't you stay-ee-ay-ee-ay*
> *Just a little bit longer . . .*

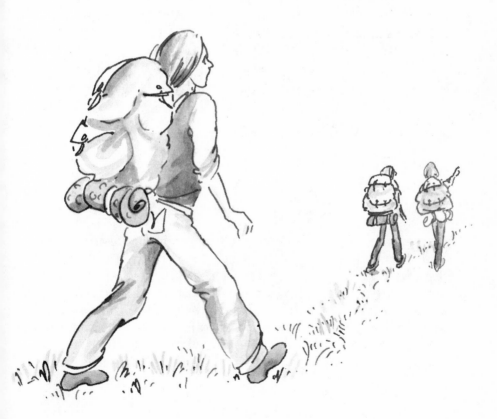

Now we head into the woods proper. Stones and roots and up and down for a couple of miles. We climb a hill that raises my pulse to 120, an equivalent in energy expenditure to a mile-long jog. At the top of the hill, we have a second breakfast, on a little platform of moss-covered rock. "A soda," says Julian, "my kingdom for a soda."

Two well-equipped walkers come in the opposite direction up the hill, the first people we've seen today. At 9:45 we're off again. Our impact on the wilderness has been self-consciously light: some cherry pits flicked into the surrounding bushes, a piece of bread that the birds will get, and some fat tipped into a small dip in the rock as an experiment to see how soon ants came (they ignored it). I carry away some empty raisin boxes to dump when we find a trash can.

As we walk, I see indications of some of the problems that beset the Appalachian Trail Conference. On either side along the road were nice country houses, with sun rooms, screens, well-mown lawns and their gardens open to anyone who wants to travel the trail. Some walkers can look pretty rough, others are perhaps less than considerate. Pasted on one of the trees was a "NO TRESPASSING" notice, perhaps the result of a bad experience with walkers. I see a similar notice on another tree –

PRIVATE LAND – OWNER ALLOWS HIKING
PLEASE RESPECT THE PRIVILEGE.

and then another:

LEAVE NO LITTER
START NO FIRES
CUT NO TREES
STAY ON THE TRAIL

All are indications of the conflict between the desires of the trail user and the rights of private ownership. The privilege of use can be withdrawn at any time. There is no legal compulsion to force landowners to give access to trail users. There is no right-of-way law to be established or re-established as there is in England. The trail must be sustained with a combination of tenacity and understanding to balance two fundamental desires: for a living wilderness open to all and for the security of private property.

Stopping to ponder over the last notice, I drop a bit behind.

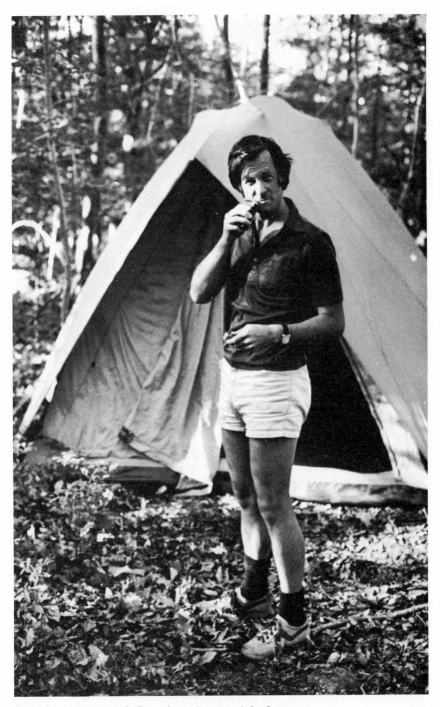

Roughing it, sort of: I can't resist a quick shave.

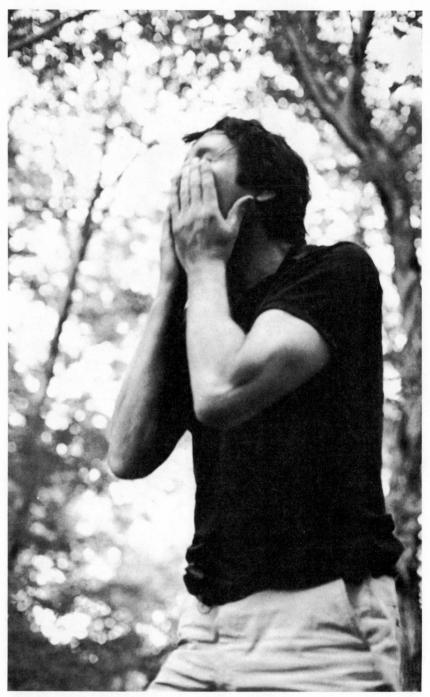

Desmond wakes himself up with a dash of cold water.

162

Hurrying to catch up, I miss the trail and head off along an overgrown track. I find myself in the depths of the wood. I am in unfamiliar territory, without map or compass. I listen to the silence. I shout. No reply. I have no idea how far back I lost the trail. Not far, but what if I fail to retrace my steps accurately? My imagination is beginning to run wild. I set off back. I pick up a white flash on a tree. A track. I turn along it. After about a quarter of a mile, as if to provide confirmation I am on the trail again, two tubby girls with Bridgeport, Connecticut, T-shirts pass me going in the other direction. I emerge on a dusty track at what looks like a school. The pangs of nervousness evaporate. Julian is waiting, unconcerned.

A sign informs us that positively no horses or dogs are allowed on the grounds; it is signed "The Sisters." It sounds a bit ominous, but I suppose it is a convent school. Desmond has walked over to the buildings to try to get some water. He returns, successful.

Off we go, on the grit track. I hear mewing from our right. It sounds very much like a cat, but in fact it's a rough grouse trying to lead us away from its nest, which must be in some ivy by the side of the road here.

We seem suddenly to be back in suburbia. Somebody has mown the side of the grass and the track has been watered to keep the dust down. For about half an hour we walk on the hard surface. You *do* get into the rhythm of it, but it's tough on the calves. I'll be glad when we get back into the woodland, which lies about half a mile ahead.

We turn off the hard road and go through what the trail guide describes as an open hardwood forest. The trees average about twenty feet apart and one can see two hundred or three hundred yards through them. The foliage makes a roof, sixty feet above us. We haven't been out in direct sunlight all morning and it occurs to me that this is a cool way to travel, shielded even at midday by a canopy of leaves.

Heading for the Old West Point road, where I guess that Desmond and Julian will head back up north somehow, leaving me to go it alone, we descend the steepest and longest slope we have met so far. It is a dried-up riverbed. In winter or fall it would be a torrent. Now it is a tangle of stones and roots, dropping down at about 45 degrees in a rough staircase of boulders, loose earth and branches. My thighs are aching. It is

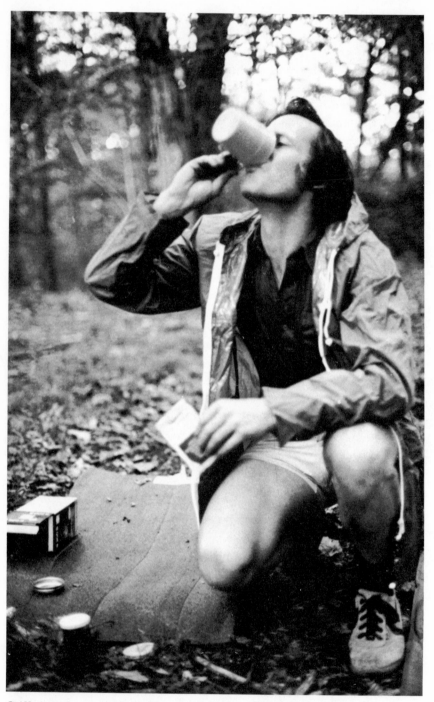

Still time for one last swig of coffee before breaking camp.

the longest mile of my life. About halfway down we come across some horse droppings, but I don't see how *anybody* could have got a horse down here.

Eventually the trail levels off. We cross a one-time meadow; now saplings perhaps five or ten years old cover it, a sign that all of this small area – like many others – is fast reverting to wilderness. The path is very overgrown. Bindweed reaches right across it. Saplings grapple with our backpacks.

About 1:00 PM we reach the first main road, Route 9A. In front of us stands the Bavarian Inn. By our reactions, anyone would think we have been walking for days. We collapse into beers and Cokes as if we had just crossed the Sahara. We are exhausted and exhilarated. I realize that there's no hope, with the slowness I travel through this country, of my reaching the Hudson the next day, let alone climbing Bear Mountain. That would be a day or two on its own, and I'm not yet fit enough to consider it.

Desmond remembers some friends with a swimming pool who live close by. We call them. They pick us up. We spend the afternoon swimming and drinking gallons of gin and tonic and Coke. Many walkers have said that one of the greatest joys of walking is arriving. Now I know what they mean.

When we reach home, we are full of the adventure. Our limbs ache, but we are elated at what we have accomplished.

"Fifteen miles," says Desmond, "I never thought it would be such hard work."

I look at the map.

"Fifteen miles?" I say, after a bit of calculation. "Do you realize that our marathon took us just *six* miles?" Cries of derision from the rest of the family.

Six miles! I can hardly believe it. How can anyone cover twenty miles a day with a pack twice as heavy . . . ?

Some do, and I am left in some awe at their strength and endurance.

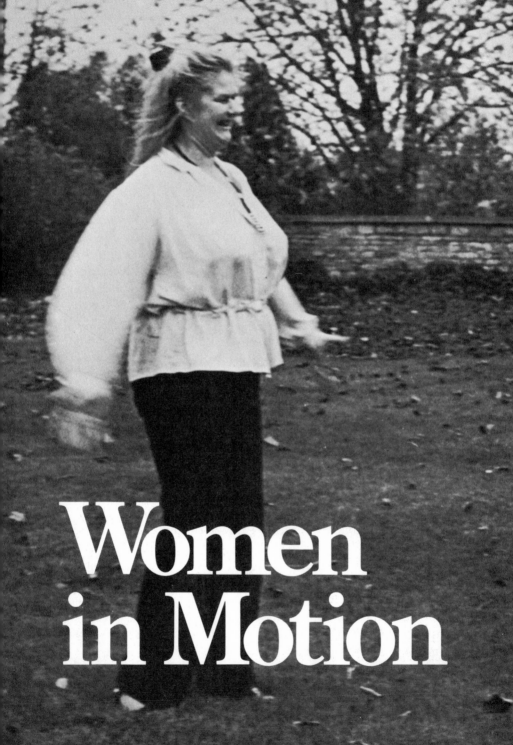

Women
in Motion

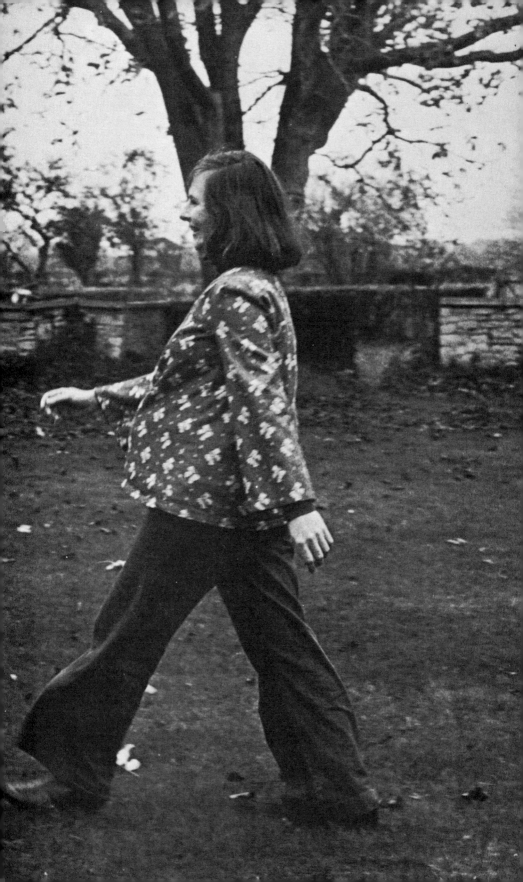

Women in Motion

ONE SPRING A FEW years ago I was vacationing in the Italian Alps with my wife Angy near Cortina d'Ampezzo, a superb skiing center cradled in the Dolomites. We decided to do some walking on the slopes. One evening we scanned a small scale map and chose a three-thousand-foot peak which seemed invitingly puny by comparison with the snow-capped giants that dominated the valley. Our map showed a little lake of melt-water near the summit and a track leading up the mountainside through the forest. Three thousand feet? We'd take a picnic, stroll up before lunch and be back by early afternoon.

Next morning we set off optimistically and found the track with no trouble. I noticed a machine that the Italians apparently used to get up the track. It was a crawler-tractor, but one built rather like a sports car. The whole thing was only about four feet high and each tread was a yard wide. The driver's cab was perched at one end. Clearly, it was designed to travel up slopes of at least 45 degrees, and rightly so: that was the angle at which the track zig-zagged up through the forest. After about a quarter of an hour, when we'd climbed no more than three hundred feet, the prospect that had seemed so charming over supper began to pall.

"Hey," I said to Angy, who for some reason seemed always to be a couple of yards ahead of me, "how about leaving it till tomorrow?"

"Don't be silly," she replied. "Now that we've started, we might as well keep going."

The logic of this remark escaped me. It was precisely because we'd begun that I wanted to give it up. However, not to be outdone, I plodded on, noticing that I was now about *five* yards behind.

In the course of the next three and a half hours, which is what it took to climb the three thousand feet, we stopped many times, always at my request. As it happened, the walk was well worth it. I saw my first marmot. The lake was beautiful. We ate in the clean, clear silence at the upper limit of the tree line. That much was predictable. What I hadn't reckoned on was my own physical incompetence. It was a painful way to learn that Angy could walk me off my feet up a mountain – and ample proof that women are, in some respects, as tough as men and occasionally even tougher.

When I began writing this book, it occurred to me that I ought to look into this and find out a couple of things about women and walking. In what ways are they different from men in physical capacity? In what ways can walking be of special importance for them?

Beneath the Myth There's Muscle

It was something of a revelation to learn just how little difference there need be between men and women in terms of muscle power and endurance. Until very recently western society did not encourage women to take exercise. Anything more than light indulgence in sport was supposed to be unladylike. I remember at college a contemporary of mine commenting on a massive Russian woman shot-putter: "What a disgusting sight! Look what happens when a woman takes up a man's sport!" I knew what he meant: exercise had put the muscle on her and men didn't like muscles on women. Women were supposed to be demure, soft and smooth. Intense physical activity tarnished this image. Let them stay as they are – "the weaker sex." And besides, didn't we all know that women were even weaker once a month? When I was a child I always heard women with their periods described as "indisposed" and, like many others before and after me, I grew up with a vague feeling that the essential fragility of women was always threatening to break through.

There have, of course, always been activities that were perfectly acceptable and which gave the lie to all these myths. Not even the most chauvinistic, beer-swilling football player would have dreamed of describing Pavlova or Fonteyn as unfeminine or overmuscular. Indeed, ballet dancing has always

169

seemed to exemplify the very essence of femininity. Ballerinas clearly have the strength and endurance and explosive power of superb athletes. And not only ballet dancers: I remember at college a high jumper, Nell Truman, sister of the tennis player Christine Truman, who weight-trained, an unusual activity for a woman two decades ago. She used to do squats with over 200 pounds on her shoulders which, given her slight 112-pound frame, indicated a power-weight ratio which many male athletes would have been proud to achieve.

It is only recently, however, that physiologists have begun to measure what the *significant* differences are between men and women. Dr. Jack Wilmore at the University of California has done some basic research on the matter. His findings indicate that up to the age of 12 there are few differences in strength and endurance between the sexes. Thereafter men become bigger and stronger, hence faster; yet the efficiency of a woman's muscles is equal to that of a man's. The mean strength of young, nonathletic women can be improved by as much as 30 percent over a ten-week training program. In leg strength, for instance, untrained women were found to be about 25 percent weaker than untrained men in absolute terms; but when leg strength was related to body weight, the differences were reduced to 7.6 percent. When the values were expressed relative to *lean* body weight – that is, muscle fiber for muscle fiber – the women actually proved to be 5.8 percent stronger. Dr. Wilmore also pointed out that women have the built-in capacity to gain strength as efficiently as men without gaining muscle weight.

In tests of endurance men and women display huge differences when untrained. But when trained, according to another study, the difference between the sexes in efficiency of oxygen uptake narrows to only 3.4 percent. Since women are generally shorter and have a higher percentage of fat, they will not, as a group, be able to rival men in endurance or speed, but in muscular efficiency they differ hardly at all from men.

These findings – combined with the fact that women are now training and competing more seriously than ever before – are reflected in the declining gap between women's records and men's. For instance, in the 1924 Olympics the winning time for men in the 400-meter free-style swimming competition was 16 percent better than the winning women's time. It is now only about 7 percent faster. In long-distance running women seem to

> *"In one respect, women are still suffering from their domestic straightjacket. They continue to be judged the physically weaker sex, and even many of the feminists choose not to context the point. Recent studies have shown, however, that this stigma may be just another culturally induced myth – one which is fostered, and in the process, confirmed by the sedentary life foisted upon most women."*
>
> Dr. Jack Wilmore, University of California

have a positive advantage conferred by their higher percentage of body fat, which seems to provide an efficient source of fuel. In one or two cases over very long distances (fifty miles and one hundred miles), women have actually performed better than men. Another stunning example is the fact that in the last ten years the women's marathon record has come down from 3 hours 15 minutes 22 seconds to 2 hours 38 minutes 19 seconds, a tremendous drop in time, while over the same period the men's marathon record has fallen by little more than a minute.

Nor is performance necessarily dependent upon the time of the month. Marje Albohn, of the Department of Health, Physical Education and Recreation at Indiana University, has summarized the relationship between menstruation and exercise in *The Physician and Sportsmedicine* magazine: "Despite the complex chemical and hormonal changes that women experience every month, the actual effect on physical performance is negligible. The blood loss during menstruation is so small that it has no measurable effect on physical capacity." Even in cases of dysmenorrhea – painful periods – "it has been shown that people in regular exercise have fewer problems."

Walking Your Way to a Healthy and Happy Pregnancy

An Interview with Britain's Sheila Kitzinger

So women can, when walking, equal their male companions in endurance. What of the benefits (or dangers) of walking during pregnancy, when women surely do need special consideration?

To answer this question, I talked with one of Britain's leading writers on pregnancy and childbirth, Sheila Kitzinger. She is a

171

perfect person to seek guidance from: in addition to being the mother of five daughters, she is enthusiastic and clear, with an expressive face and physique that she uses with flamboyance to dramatize her words. She is, quite simply, exhilarating to talk to, especially for someone as unfamiliar as I was with her ideas.

"Walking is far better than traditional prenatal exercises," she told me. "Take straight-leg lifting, one of the old stand-bys. The woman lies down flat on her back and then lifts one leg straight, then the other leg straight and then both legs straight. The idea is to strengthen her abdominal muscles, but in fact, what she is really doing is putting terrific stress on her lower spine and on the rectus muscle, down the front. In advanced pregnancy, the abdominal contents can actually press out through the divided rectus muscle."

I suggested that it seemed unnatural to lie on one's back and wave one's legs in the air.

"If you look at traditional prenatal exercises as a whole," she went on, "you'll see that there is an entire range of these activities that are 'unnatural' and don't relate to normal movement. Many of them are really physical jerks, nonrhythmical movements which are not only stressful to some women, but also potentially positively harmful. There's another exercise which involves the woman getting down on all fours and humping her back up as high as she can while dropping her head, then hollowing her back and raising her head. This is probably perfectly all right for most people. But a proportion of women often develop acute backache during pregnancy (associated with slackened ligaments), and if they do this exercise, they may make their backache much worse."

I remembered Angy doing a good deal of breathing and relaxation exercises. "What about these?" I asked.

"Some of those exercises are just plain pointless. There are certain relaxation exercises supposed to help body awareness, which involve contracting all the muscles of the right arm [*she tensed it dramatically*] . . . and then dropping the arm [*she let it collapse back into her chair*] . . . contracting all the muscles of the left arm [*tense*] . . . and dropping the arm [*collapse*]; right leg; left leg; right leg *and* left arm, and so on. All of this doesn't really help a woman to get on better terms with her body. It bears absolutely no relation to the sort of psychosomatic co-ordination that she's going to need in labor. Yet that was one of

172

the basic exercises of psychoprophylaxis, and it's still being taught by some childbirth educators. Even the breathing exercises often taught in prenatal classes are sometimes too forced, involving a great sucking in of air, which prepares a woman to overbreathe and, in turn, to flush out carbon-dioxide from her bloodstream.

"It's much better to move and breathe naturally. What's important is to exercise the *whole* body, keep the circulation going, pump oxygen to the body. This is why walking is so marvelous. So is belly dancing, which is an extension of walking. The right sort of breathing occurs quite naturally when you do that sort of movement. If you're sitting down, it's very difficult to lift the ribcage properly when the baby is high up under the ribs toward the end of pregnancy. You need to be up and moving to get the ribcage free.

"In late pregnancy a woman may find herself breathing more rapidly and lightly because she cannot breathe deeply. She shouldn't feel that she must do complete breaths all the time. But if she walks briskly – not just strolls, but swings her arms and gets a good pelvic movement going – then she'll find herself spontaneously breathing just that little bit deeper."

I asked about circulation problems.

"Surprisingly, this is sometimes a problem around the vulva itself and around the rectum. Varicose veins of the vulva and hemorrhoids can be nasty. And, of course, varicose veins in the legs are quite common. Again mobilization is the answer. Movement pumps the blood back to the heart much more effectively than if the woman is still. In fact, a pregnant woman should never stand around. She should always move. Even if she's at a cocktail party and she doesn't find it easy to move, she should at least be walking on the spot every now and again."

But should one really be walking at all with all that weight to carry around?

"Yes, yes. But so many of us do it incorrectly. There's a very exaggerated sacro-lumbar curve in late pregnancy. The shape of the woman's lower spine actually changes. Whereas before it was almost straight, now the bit at the very back of the pelvis becomes more concave. This happens quite naturally. There's nothing wrong with it. But it means that a woman has to adjust her balance.

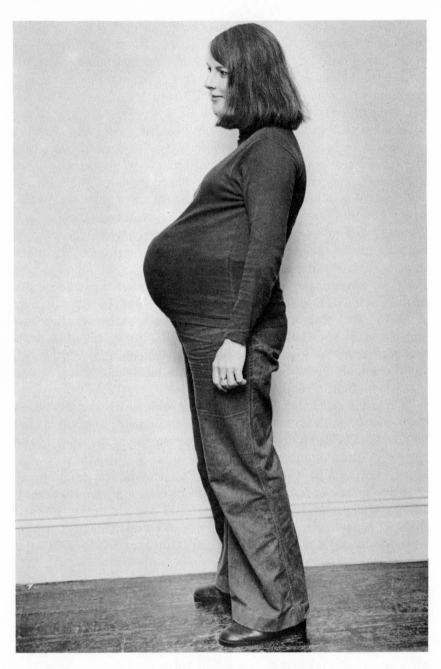

Nyree Parsonage, two weeks before she gave birth to a baby girl, demonstrates a classic slouched pose with shoulders drooping backward and stomach pushed forward—exactly the kind of posture that leads to lower and upper backache in so many pregnant women.

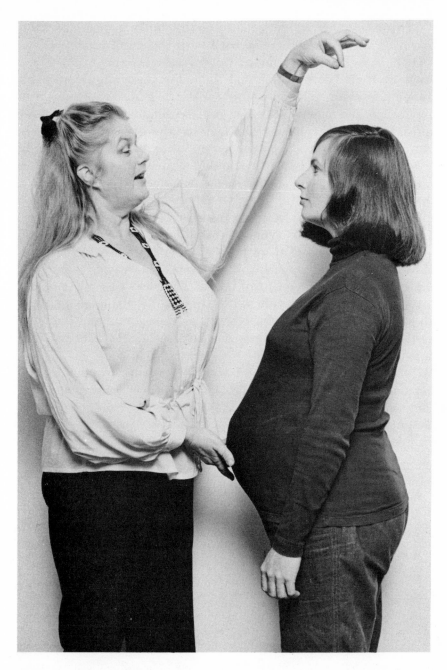

Sheila Kitzinger shows her how to correct her slouch and get her body into alignment by telling her to imagine that the crown of her head is being pulled upward while at the same time she tucks her hips under the baby.

"Think of the weight of the baby pulling her abdomen forward. Many women try to cope with the sacro-lumbar curve and the weight of the baby by hollowing the back still further, sticking their bottoms out and throwing their shoulders back in compensation. They develop a sort of waddle. . . . [*She got to her feet, planted her toes apart and began to move laboriously across the room, splaying her legs as she did so.*] The extraordinary thing is they not only get lower backache, but they get it high up behind their shoulders as well, and they often can't understand why. It's because they've tried to cope with the extra weight by flinging their shoulders back."

"*So?*" I prompted. "*How can you correct this?*"

"Well, the trick is to avoid trying to do all the work with your abdominal muscles. You're just making extra work for them, because it can't be done from the front. The way to cope with the weight is to tuck your tail under. That way you lift the baby into the cradle of your pelvis. It's almost like lifting an egg into an eggcup, if you think of the pelvis as the eggcup and the baby as the egg. Then you can use the natural girdle of abdominal muscle quite spontaneously.

"It's easiest to get the right walking posture by tucking the buttocks together like two tight little buns. This way the buttock muscles can act as reinforcements to hold the added weight in the pelvis securely. A good way to get the feel of it is

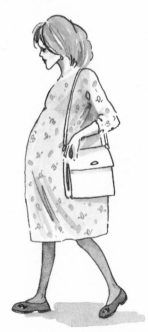

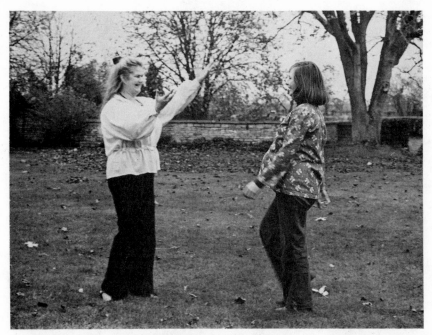

Under Sheila's energetic direction, Nyree strides out at a pace sufficient to ensure muscular strength and good circulation, bringing benefits to both baby and mother-to-be.

to imagine that you have a $10 bill between your buttocks and somebody's trying to take it away from you. No one can walk around like that all the time, of course, but it's an easy way to give you the feeling of it. And if a pregnant woman does that in front of a full-length mirror, sideways on, she'll notice the change in her profile. She can often look two months less pregnant. Once she's found the right posture she'll find that her legs swing naturally from the pelvis with their normal pendulum motion. The splayed Donald Duck waddle vanishes. And if she remembers to swing her shoulders, she'll even get rid of any upper back pain she's had."

We then went on to discuss how and where one walks and what to wear.

"I think one has to make a distinction between different types of walking," she said. "It should not be strolling from one shop to another. It should not take place in an atmosphere loaded with carbon-monoxide. Ideally, it should take place in the countryside or in a park or even a yard. And I think, if possible, it should be on grass rather than on hard pavement.

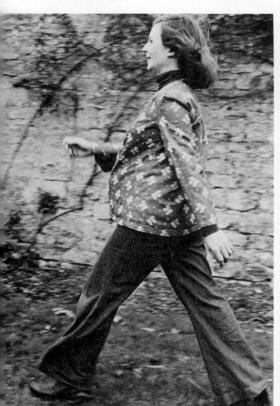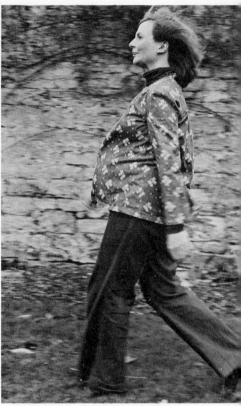

"Shoes are also important. A 1½-inch heel is ample height for a pregnant woman's shoes, and many women prefer to wear sandals or flat shoes. But if a woman's not used to flat shoes, she may only be comfortable if she has a heel. The main thing is to wear what's comfortable.

"Dress? Obviously it must be fairly loose fitting. Pregnant women tend to have their own central-heating arrangements; they get very hot very quickly, so cotton is good, because you don't want to finish your walk sweaty and exhausted. The important thing, though, is to be happy with what you're wearing."

By now I was aware of my own appalling ignorance, and was happy to do no more than insert the occasional diffident question. Sheila was way ahead of me.

"Now there's another side to all this I have to tell you about: the benefits of walking to the unborn baby." *I nodded. Of*

178

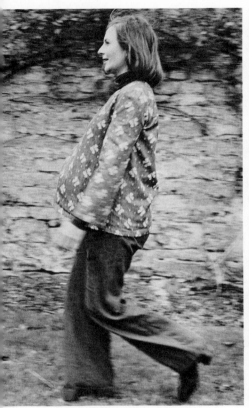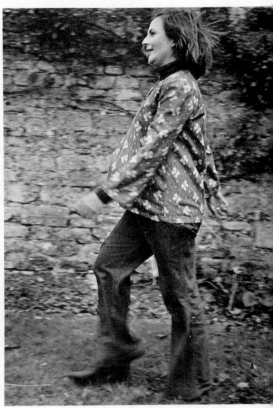

course, tell me. "The pelvis is like a cradle to the baby. Every rhythmic walking movement involves a pelvic rock, from front to back. Walking rocks the cradle in which the baby is lying.

"You can test the effect quite easily by placing your fingers on those big bones at the front of the pelvis and then tucking the tail in and slightly hollowing the back as in a walking movement. Now this is important for the baby. There have been studies done on the soothing effect of different sorts of rocking on newborn babies and it has been demonstrated that babies are most contented when the speed and motion of rocking is the equivalent of a slow walk. It's no coincidence. The motion of walking and the motion of rocking are one and the same thing. If a woman walks regularly in pregnancy and then walks with her baby slung against her body once it is born, she is giving valuable continuity to her baby's experience – the security and comfort of a rhythmic movement that it already knew when it

179

The Ambrose Effect

After speaking to Sheila Kitzinger, I called on Dr. Tony Ambrose, the doctor who pioneered the studies on rocking that Sheila had mentioned.

"I was trying to find a way of soothing babies," he told me. "I tried every sort of rocking speed and motion, from 10 times to 100 times a minute. I found that there was an ideal: 60 rocks per minute – one per second, the speed of a slow walk – with a vertical measurement of $2\frac{3}{4}$ inches. I should emphasize I'm not talking about the normal swaying rock as in a cradle, but an up-and-down motion. At this amplitude, all babies – except hungry ones – stopped crying within 15 seconds."

"Why?"

"I've no idea. But it's common knowledge that babies carried by their mothers cry less. That's the natural state of affairs. What's unnatural for a baby is to lie isolated in a clean, healthy crib, deprived of parental and environmental stimulation. I think the Ambrose Effect is something to do with the way babies sense movement – with the inner ear – and the reaction to it of the nervous system. The effect should therefore be the same on unborn babies."

---

was inside her body. The result is a contented baby."

After a walk is there any special way the expectant mother should rest?

"Yes, after walking – or working – of course she needs rest. But lying on her back can be a problem. With the enlarged uterus, the weight of the baby and the weight of the placenta, there's a pressure on the inferior vena cava (the largest vein in the abdomen) and this reduces the flow of blood – and thus oxygen – through the placenta to the baby. So she should either lie on her side, or be on a couch or in an easy chair with her feet up or in bed with lots of pillows behind. She shouldn't lie flat. Indeed, many women are so uncomfortable that they spontaneously prefer not to lie flat because they get nauseous or dizzy."

That seemed to be about it. But Sheila was still going strong.

"Don't you want to know about walking during labor?" she asked.

Walking during labor? From what I'd seen of labor, women couldn't possibly walk. What an extraordinary idea!

"No, it's not extraordinary at all. It's done all over the world. Thirty or forty years ago all midwives got their patients to walk during the first stage of labor and kept them walking for as long as they could because they wanted gravity to help them. The idea was to produce pressure from the baby's head against the cervix, and then guide the baby down the cervical canal. It's the idea of *not* walking that's revolutionary. And the awful thing is that it's been introduced accidentally, as a by-product of modern obstetric care. We've changed from birth at home to birth in the hospital. Hospital patients are supposed to be tucked neatly into bed. Many hospitals wouldn't know what to do with expectant mothers who walked around. They'd embarrass everybody. And, of course, the modern technology of labor – the medication, the monitoring systems and so on – all continue to immobilize women. If a woman's been knocked out with Demerol (pethidine), then certainly she'll be in bed because she may be rather unsafe if she's walking around. And obviously a woman can't walk after she's had a spinal epidural or any form of regional anesthesia."

But in traditional home births, what happens if you're walking around and you have a contraction?

"Then you stop and lean against something. You lean against the wall, or a shelf, or a piece of furniture, or your husband, or your sister, or your mother."

What's the point? Is there any indication that a contraction would be easier to deal with?"

"Oh, yes. Women are much better able to tolerate powerful contractions when they're upright and walking around. The contractions are more effective than when the mother is lying down, but she doesn't feel them as much. The whole thing's much better, the fetal heart is much more regular, and labor is shorter."

How long can it continue?

"There is no reason why a woman shouldn't keep moving, if she wishes, until she delivers. In some California communes, women in labor are encouraged to do lots of movement during not only the first, but also the second stage of labor. This is actually quite appropriate. A large proportion of labors, perhaps about a third of them, are backache labors, caused by the baby facing the mother's front rather than toward her back, so that the hard part of the baby's head is really pressing against

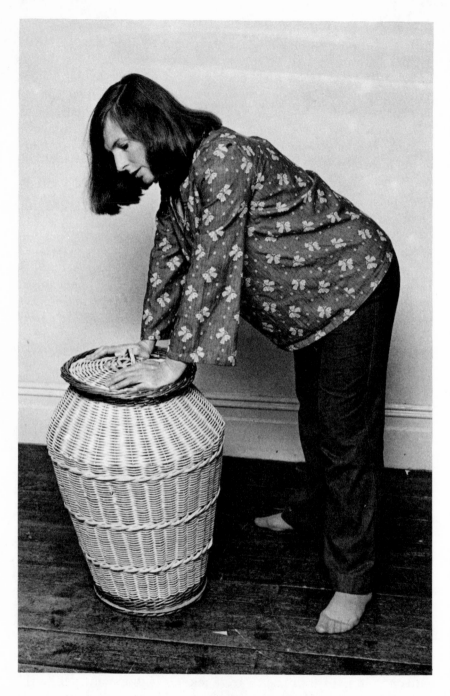

A correct position for easing a contraction while walking during labor: stop and lean yourself against something.

Walk! It Could Ease Your Labor

A report in the British Medical Journal *(August 26, 1978) entitled "Ambulation in Labor" studied the effects of walking during labor on a group of thirty-four women who were monitored continuously.*

Uterine action was significantly better. . . . The first stage of labor from the time of monitoring or ambulation was over two hours shorter in the ambulant group than in the group nursed in bed. More of the patients nursed in bed needed augmentation of labor. Contractions were less frequent and the amplitude greater in the ambulant group.

The ambulant patients needed less analgesia: twenty patients needed neither pethidine (Demerol) nor an epidural analgesic. The mean dose in patients who did need analgesia was also smaller among those who were ambulant. The fetal heart rate patterns show the beneficial effects of ambulation on the fetus and the newborn.

We would agree that the nursing of the ambulant patient in labor is different, but it is not more complicated, and continuous monitoring using radiotelemetry is not a problem.

The advantages to the mother and her fetus indicate that ambulation in labor should be encouraged. The beneficial effects might be due to the labor being more natural, the effect of gravity, or the reduced need for analgesia and augmentation, or a combination of all three.

---

the sacrum. This occipito-posterior position, as it is called, often results in the most excruciating backache, which goes on between, as well as during, contractions. The worst possible thing you can do to a woman then is to make her lie down in bed on her back, because she would have the whole weight of the baby against her back. It also gives the baby's head less of a chance to rotate into the right position because the mother has wedged it into a difficult position. Spontaneously, she'll try to get up or roll over onto her side, and either of these positions can allow the baby to rotate into the right position better. In short, the important thing with a backache labor is to get the baby's weight off the spine. And the best way of doing this is walking."

And what about walking after the birth?

"It's dangerous for the woman to lie in bed after delivering. There's a risk of thrombosis. So I'm all for the principle of early ambulation. In England a woman is ambulant normally six hours after delivery. Of course, if she's had a regional anesthesia or an episiotomy (which in the US is an almost automatic procedure in 98 out of 100 deliveries), she may not quite be ready. But if she is ready, it seems best for her to get up slowly from her bed; swing her legs over the side; sit for a moment on the bed to make sure that her circulation is working well and that she's not going to get giddy; get up; tuck her buttocks together, because there's an enormous readjustment of weight; and then walk slowly, in a serene way, as soon after childbirth as she feels able to. For some women, that would be, oh, half an hour – perhaps as little as ten minutes – after delivery.

"Thereafter, walking can be beneficial both for breast feeding and for rehabilitation. One of the main problems encountered for lactating women nowadays is stasis of milk. The first signs of stasis is a red patch on the breast, often appearing in the outer quadrant. This simply means that the milk is not getting down into the nipple and is producing an inflamed spot on the breast. I have seen this happening when a woman is sitting or lying around and not getting up and about and moving her arms. If it is not treated, it can lead to mastitis (inflammation of the breast) and even, in some cases, to breast abscess. It's most likely to happen when a woman thinks: I must have rest! Everybody's telling me I need rest! I won't be able to nurse properly unless I have rest!

"But for a sound, natural cure, you only have to think of peasant women all over the world: they breast feed far more successfully than we do, and yet they can't possibly have the kind of rest which we are often prescribed after childbirth. They've got to go on stirring the cooking pot and rubbing the clothes on the stones down by the river and carrying water urns. The answer lies in vigorous arm movement. One of the first treatments for stasis is energetic arm movements, and one of the best energetic arm movements is wringing out diapers. But how many women do that nowadays? We've got paper ones and diaper liners and so on. Another good exercise is polishing a floor on your hands and knees, but again who does it?

"This is precisely where walking comes in. My advice to any couple is usually to buy a baby carrier, go out and walk together

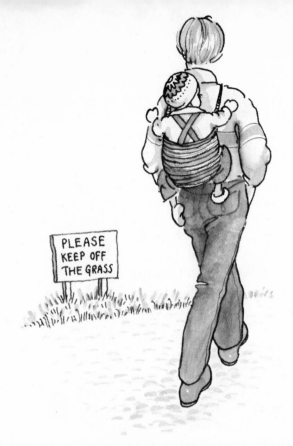

with your baby. It's not only good for the baby; it's good for the mother."

It seems like walking is something of a wonder cure. What other effects does it have on the new mother?

"It's also a tremendous help for other parts of the body. Of course, if there's been an episiotomy, recovery is a long, slow process. But healthy movement in the form of walking can increase elasticity of the tissues, provided the woman doesn't get overtired and exhausted.

"Finally, we've got to think of the muscle of the pelvic floor, one of the most important parts of a woman's body. Think of holding a soapy sponge as you lie in the bath. The soap fills all the little holes in the sponge. Now, the more the sponge is squeezed and released, the more the soap will go out and the fresh water – the blood – will come in. After childbirth, very often, this pelvic muscle is bruised and tender, and the more difficult the labor, the more it is bruised.

"Many women almost cut themselves off from the problem. They leave that part of their bodies for the obstetricians to

---

*"A walk: the air incredibly pure, delights for the eye, a warm
and gently caressing sunlight, one's whole being joyous."*
Henri Frederic Amiel, *What a Lovely Walk!*

---

worry about. They don't want anything to do with it. It still
isn't quite their own again. And so they don't exercise this part
of the body.

"Yet I can't stress enough how important it is to remember
that the more a muscle is tightened, held firm for a little while
and then released, tightened, held and released again, the more
you get fresh oxygenated blood flowing in which aids rehabilitation. After childbirth, a woman should be doing this regularly
when she's out walking, when she goes up and down stairs and
when she's doing housework. It can be linked with chores like
changing diapers, but it's better for a woman to have regular
exercise out of doors and for her to do this rhythmic contrac-
tion-release-contraction-release as she moves. It fits in quite
spontaneously with regular walking movements.

"Ideally, a woman, when she's walking, should have her
pelvic floor muscles in the shape of a smile. Our pelvic muscles
reflect our moods, in a way. We don't go around with our
mouths sagging. The pelvic floor needs to do exactly the same.
It has a lot to do, holding up all the pelvic contents and hence at
one remove all the abdominal contents."

*I didn't want her to stop there. "What of menopause?" I asked,
"do you think walking can help there?"*

"In the traditional, tribal experience, growing older confers
new benefits on a woman. Exactly the opposite seems to happen
now in Western societies. Many women feel in spite of themselves and in spite of what they tell themselves, intellectually,
that they're no longer needed in the same way. And this has its
effect on a woman's whole body tissue, on her muscles, on the
way she uses them, and certainly on the way she walks. The
effect is especially powerful on her pelvic muscles, which
begin to sag. Collapse of the spirit leads to physical collapse – in
particular to prolapse (or, a falling down) of the uterus. We
can't simply see a prolapse in isolated, mechanical terms. It's
something to do with the woman's relationship with her body,

186

the way she feels about her body and the normal posture, the normal good posture or bad posture of invisible muscles in her body.

"The exciting thing is that this is not final. A woman who has lost her physical and emotional well-being can usually reverse the process if she exercises – even a woman in her 70s. Mind and body are interdependent.

"A woman who has confidence and trust in herself and is able to live through and express herself with her body instead of just seeing it as an encumbrance is healthy. It seems to me that at any stage in a woman's life, walking should be a natural part of her everyday life."

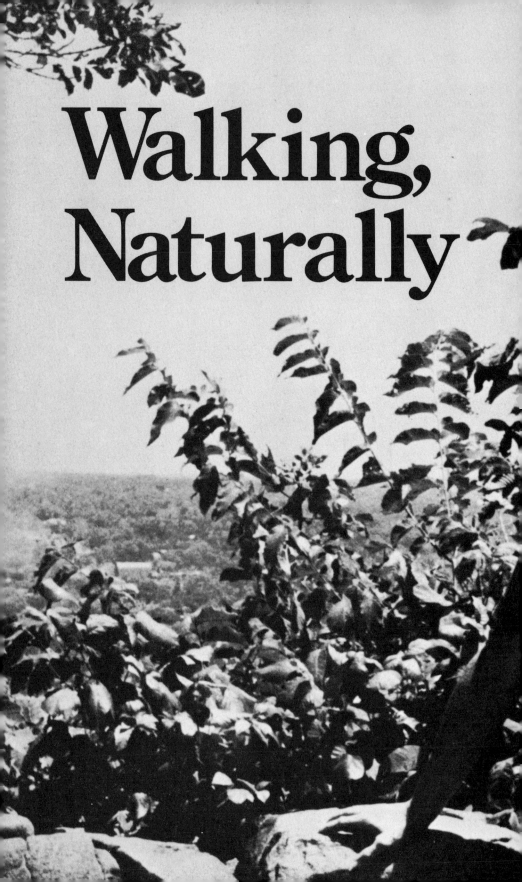

Walking, Naturally

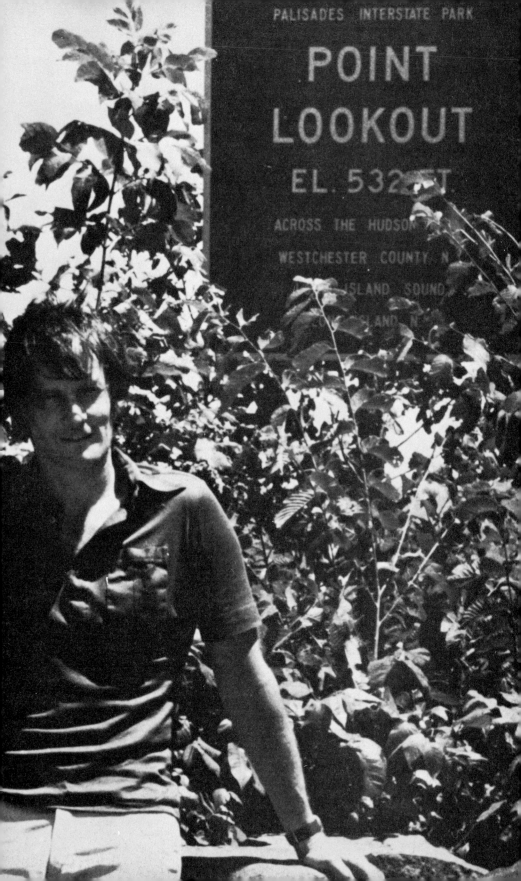

PALISADES INTERSTATE PARK

POINT
LOOKOUT

EL. 532 FT

ACROSS THE HUDSON

WESTCHESTER COUNTY, N

ISLAND SOUND

LAND, N

Walking, Naturally

GOOD HEALTH IS NOT simply a matter of physical well-being in combination with the mental relaxation that exercise brings. Most people with a vigorous hobby like to bring to it some positive mental activity. Some runners have a passion for the achievements of others and become wizards at statistics. Golfers can become obsessed with the intricacies of woods and plastics. As a walker I get particular pleasure out of seeking explanations for the look, shape and feel of the landscape around me. One cannot, of course, nature walk all the time. It is essentially a slow occupation. Sometimes you have to stand and watch, or sit and use your imagination. And to get the best out of a nature walk – unless you are yourself an expert – you need some sort of guide, someone who can see beyond the surface of rocks and leaves and explain to you the hidden dimensions of the scenery. The few occasions on which I have had the benefit of a knowledgeable guide have proved revelations. The information I have picked up on these brief but intense walks is now a latticework into which I can build experiences of other walks in similar environments.

A Walk through Time

Soon after I first arrived in New York a number of years ago, I became involved in the production of a book on the natural history of New York City. The work set me wondering. I was puzzled by the shape of the place. To the east and south lie soft, sweeping Atlantic beaches, backed by Long Island's well-rounded hills and by reedy marshlands. A few miles away towers Manhattan, the skyscrapers offering visible evidence of the solidity of the underlying rock fabric. Westward and northward, fringing the Hudson for several miles, stand the

"Walkers acquire a special ownership of roads and streets and parks and fields."

Hal Borland, *To Own the Streets and Fields*

imposing five-hundred foot stockade-like slabs of rock called the Palisades. Why are these three distinct features so close together?

To answer this question I turned again to New York geologist Sid Horenstein of the Museum of Natural History. An expert in local geology, he looks at the sands, hills, cliffs and tumbled boulders in and around New York with a proprietary passion and never tires of attempting to infuse newcomers with his enthusiasm. He is a great publicist for geology – and an avid walker.

Sid and I went on a number of walks together. They took us, in turn, to the seaside sanctuary of Jamaica Bay just by Kennedy Airport, to the northern tip of Manhattan, to the Palisades, and to the Great Swamp, a small wildlife reserve in New Jersey, thirty miles west of Manhattan.

First then to Jamaica Bay, which looks like a large freshwater lake dotted with rushy islands, rich in bird life. Along one side runs the border of JFK Airport. Hazy in the distance stand the monolithic towers of the World Trade Center. The bay's twelve thousand acres form the world's largest wildlife refuge within the confines of a city. Surprisingly, it is an artificial sanctuary. The bay was once open to the sea, but in the 1930s and '40s, as the city's patchwork of streets and airports crowded out toward the coast, wilderness lovers argued increasingly strongly that the bay should be protected. In the 1950s the Transit Authority proposed to rebuild the railroad that ran across the middle of the bay. They were given permission to do so by the city's Parks Commissioner, Robert Moses, but only on condition that they build dikes to feed in fresh water and thus create a new environment. In 1953 the bay was established as a wildlife refuge.

Over the next twenty years the first superintendant, Herb Johnson, had the sandy islands stabilized with a variety of grasses which, in combination with new trees and shrubs, now attract some three hundred species of birds every year. Occa-

191

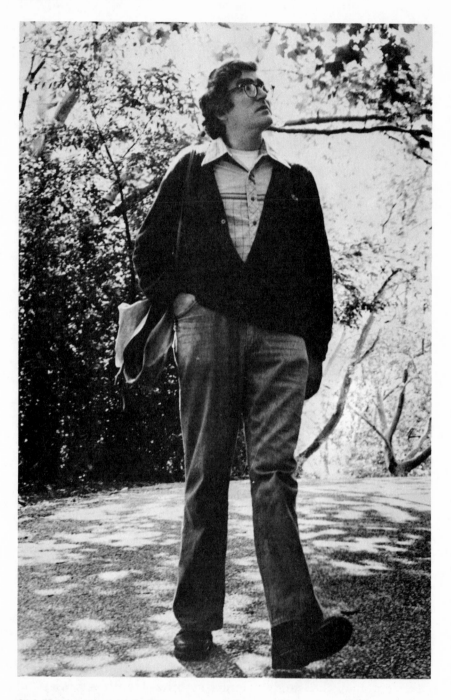

Sid Horenstein, geologist, nature walker and New York City walker extraordinaire.

sionally, "birders" – and there must have been thirty or forty on watch when we were there – are rewarded with a real rarity. In 1959, for instance, they recorded the arrival of a European red-winged thrush which had never been seen in North America before.

But Sid and I were not there to look at wildlife that day. "See the city?" he said with a sweep of his arm. "You can imagine it as the sheer edge of a plateau, can't you? Well, ten thousand years ago, roughly along that line, there *was* a plateau: ice. Except that it was a good bit higher than those high-rise buildings. No ice here, though," and he turned to look east and west.

"We're standing just beyond the reach of the last great ice sheet. That leading edge was like a huge bulldozer blade, scraping and pushing top soil from the north, and this is where it dumped it. Long Island is the terminal moraine of an ice-age glacier, cut through in some places – perhaps just here was one of them – by rivers of melted ice."

It was an imposing piece of information, one that altered my attitude somewhat to the suburban wastes of Queens. The expressways, the groups of apartment houses and cheek-to-cheek houses suddenly seemed like a minor modification of the long-term patterns of the earth's history.

Next Sid took me to the northern tip of Manhattan, to Inwood Hill, a knot of forest covering a rocky, two-hundred-foot mound that forms an unexpectedly restful retreat not far from the center of New York. A road leads to the top and there are meadows where graceful colonial mansions once stood. But the rocks have been untouched for thousands of years and the forest, in many spots, is as primeval as it was when Henry Hudson arrived in 1609 and had a minor skirmish with the resident Indians.

"These rocks," Sid told me, "are at least five hundred million

---

"It has been amusing to watch New York, which is hardly in other ways hesitant, waken by degrees to the idea that as a center for exercise on foot she may claim variety and advantage and adventure surpassed by few cities."

The New York Walk Book

---

years old. They were laid down as sediment at the bottom of a tropical sea. Then they were contorted by the shifting continents and raised many hundreds of feet into the air. Now those mountains have been cut down to mere hillocks by erosion."

"What about the Palisades, then?" I asked, "why haven't they been cut down?"

"No time," Sid replied. "They're relatively new. The Hudson over there is not only a physical barrier; it's a geological barrier and a chronological one as well. Those cliffs are volcanic and they're a mere 250 million years old. Newcomers."

Later the same week we drove north and turned west onto the George Washington Bridge, slung like a drawbridge across the Hudson to the impressive bulwarks of the Palisades. We parked near the top of the cliffs and set out along one of the many paths.

It was a magical day, the sky crisp, clear and blue with a thick carpet of autumn leaves rustling beneath the oaks, maples, hickories and dogwoods that blanket the plateau. We emerged at a magnificent vantage point, four hundred feet above the river, where one can stand like an explorer, silent before a vista stretching perhaps thirty miles north to beyond the two-mile-long Tappan Zee Bridge and south toward the city, wreathed then, as it often is, in a dome of sulfurous yellow. Hundreds of feet below me the fallen detritus of centuries – boulders, rocks and earth on which trees had scrabbled precarious root holds – sloped down and away toward the river. "Quite a height," I remarked, peering perilously out over the cliffs as near to the edge as I dared to go.

"High?" replied Sid. "Sure, but it was once much higher. When this sheet of rock was formed it was below ground. It is what's known as an igneous intrusion – volcanic rock that was once molten and forced by subterranean pressures between other, preexisting rocks. Now the overburden has been torn away, and the river has chopped off the end of the intrusion to form these cliffs. The volcanic rock began to ooze into position about 200 million years ago. As it cooled, it shrank and cracked, and it was this process that created these vertical shafts of rock."

"So there was no ice up here during the ice age?" I ventured.

"Sure there was," said Sid. "Some geologists think the ice

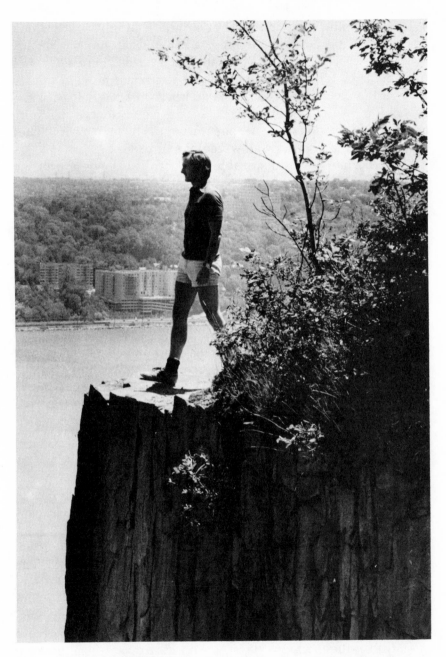

The not-so-intrepid author standing warily on a pillar of igneous rock several hundred feet sheer above the Hudson River on the Palisades, a few miles north of New York City, with a view across to the rounded, rocky hills of lower New York State, many millions of years older than the Palisades.

195

sheet was half a mile thick. That's quite a weight of ice. Look here –" and he pointed to some parallel scratches on flat exposed rock. "This is all the evidence you need. These scratches were made by rocks born along by the ice. Who knows? Perhaps they're the same ones that were dumped on Long Island. Anyway these scratches were never very deep and they're still here now, after ten thousand, perhaps fifteen thousand years. That gives you an idea of how slow geological processes are."

Slow, perhaps, but inexorable. We strolled down a winding track to the base of the cliffs. As we walked, Sid told me that the slope, known as a talus, was the product of millions of years of erosion. As frost and rain dug away at the cliffs above, the boulders tumbled down to form the heap that at some points now reaches halfway up the cliffs. "In another few million years," Sid commented, "all that will be left of the cliffs is a ridge of rock at the top of a hill."

Our fourth walk was through a place totally different in character, New Jersey's Great Swamp. The swamp lies in a basin of low hills seven miles long by three miles wide. Six thousand acres of it – almost all – is a national wildlife refuge without buildings or roads. The only way to see it is to walk.

When I first read of the place, it did not seem an exciting prospect. Much of it is underwater, turned to a poisonous-looking brown by tannins leeched from decaying vegetation. But I hadn't banked on the swamp's administrators. After we drove to the swamp and parked, somewhat to my relief Sid pointed out that there was a boardwalk specially designed to give walkers an inside view of the swamp without them ever getting their feet wet.

The swamp is something of a rarity. Wetlands are vulnerable areas; they tend to get drained, filled and paved over. The Great Swamp nearly went the same way. In 1959 the Port of New York Authority declared it was the only place it could think of to build a new metropolitan airport, but local communities banded together to buy enough of the swamp to create a wildlife refuge, which they then handed over to the government.

The swamp is a strange, brooding place. As we padded along on the planks a few inches above the brackish water, Sid told me how it came to be there. "Remember the ice age?" he said.

"Once again we're just on the edge of where the ice stopped about ten thousand years ago. We're in a bit of a hollow here, so the area was never an out-wash plain. Instead, the melt waters were caught by the surrounding hills, the Watchungs and the Ramapos. The melt water made a big lake right over all this area, some two hundred feet deep. It was here for thousands of years until the lake found an exit, through the Watchungs, along the present course of the Passaic River. The Great Swamp is almost all that's left of that lake – a remnant puddle of the ice age."

Conversations like these with Sid and others have permanently changed the spirit in which I walk. I have climbed the summit of Mount Cadillac on Mount Desert Island, Maine, and found myself reflecting on the infinitely slow collision between the American and European Continental Plates that half a billion years ago thrust the Appalachians up into towering peaks as high as the Himalayas. The 1,500-foot hillock on which I stood was the eroded core of a once majestic peak.

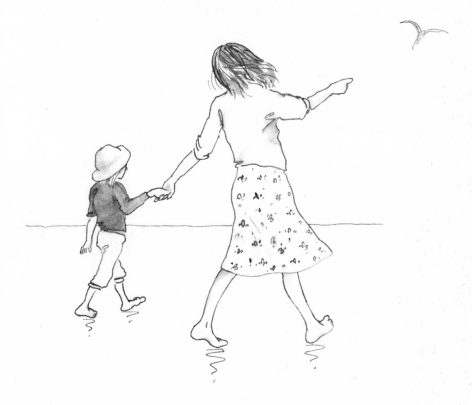

I can no longer walk the hills of Oxford without seeing the whole area as the swampy inlet of an ocean covering much of northern Europe, for that is what it was 150 million years ago. On the reedy shores, over toward London, dinosaurs roamed (the earliest known and identified dinosaur bones were found just north of Oxford; they belonged to a *Megalosaurus* that had been buried in sediment at the edge of this inlet).

I have only walked in the Alps once, but their angular steepness reminded me of how young they are geologically speaking, the result of the continuing collision between Africa and Europe, that began less than 100 million years ago.

On the Nature Trail

Thus began my awareness of one end of the chronological spectrum of the natural world, a spectrum which ranges from the mists of the geological past to the day-to-day and minute-to-minute life of animals and plants. To gain an insight into natural history of this type demands an expertise of a different sort. I can think of no better way to learn about nature than by walking a nature trail – a walk specially designed to provide such insights. Sometimes there's a guide to accompany you; usually you can use an annotated pamphlet telling you what to look out for. In the United States there are particularly superb facilities provided in the more than sixty-three sanctuaries of the National Audubon Society, named after the naturalist painter John James Audubon. Several of these sanctuaries operate as nature centers or ecology workshops and offer superb walks led by people who dispense their knowledge with enthusiasm.

I was keen to see how much it was possible to get out of a walk in an Audubon sanctuary with a trained guide, so one summer afternoon while staying in Connecticut with some friends, I headed for the Audubon Center in Greenwich, a rolling 477-acre wilderness in miniature, complete with hardwood forest, lake and swampland.

As soon as I arrived, I knew that I was in for a busy afternoon. In search of my guide, Jean Porter, I strolled into the center's reception area. Literature seemed to blossom from a hundred bookcases. There were pamphlets on the changing seasons and on the plants, flowers, birds and animals of the

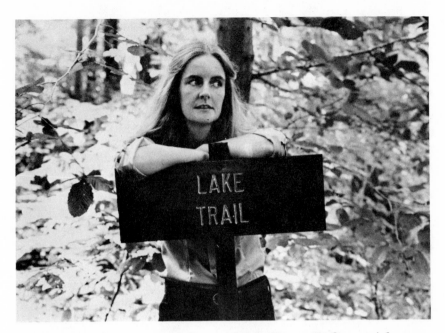

Jean Porter, nature guide at the Audubon Center in Greenwich, Connecticut.

area. There were, I learned, eighty-seven species of bird nesting in the sanctuary. The list of ferns and flowering plants was the result of an eight-year study. It seemed as if an army of naturalists must spend their lives there combing the area. There was even a monthly record of the birds that had been spotted, the most recent reporting on "what will undoubtedly be one of the most unusual and exciting sightings in our area this year . . . a Yellow Rail skulk[ing] through a goldenrod and raspberry patch." I suddenly felt overwhelmed by so much detail and was glad that I had an expert guide to point out items of significance during the walk.

Jean was a slim, trim, sun-browned blue-jeaned woman in her late 20s. She seemed everything an outdoors person should be: direct, knowledgeable and fit.

"Our fifteen miles of trails offer challenges to people of just about any physical capabilities," she explained as we set out. "There are some easy walks and there are also some fairly tough ones. And there's a variety of habitats – a lake, a stream, a small pond, a maple swamp, upland deciduous forest and overgrown pasture."

"You must know it pretty well," I ventured.

"Sure, but a lot of people are surprised to find out how much time a naturalist actually spends behind a desk. A lot of my time is spent in program planning and teaching. In fact, it's a luxury for me to get out on the trails."

The sanctuary had not always been wild. A family called Mead settled the area in the eighteenth century and established first a potato farm and later a charcoal business.

"Charcoal mounds still push through the leaves," Jean said, as we walked away from the headquarters. "You see that cottonwood tree? It was planted at the time the house was built. Magnificent, isn't it?"

There are still a few other reminders of the graceful Mead estate. We came to another almost at once – an orchard of rangy, abandoned apple trees.

"They have not been managed recently and unless we do something soon, they are going to fall over. They still bear fruit, though."

Jean led me into the woodland and then stopped short.

"Here's a vernal – a temporary – pool," she said. I didn't see much of anything, except some dried mud and a few leaves. "It's very active in the spring and is used heavily by wood frogs and toads. It dries up in the summer, so the only animals that use it to breed are ones whose strategies are for very quick tadpolehood and an immediate emergence onto land as frogs."

I liked that word: tadpolehood.

"Of course it would be a cemetary for a green frog or a bullfrog, for instance. They both spend as much as three years in the tadpole stage."

There was a scattering of leaves close by. A chipmunk.

"It's a good year for chipmunks," Jean remarked, as it scampered over the leaves, chattering. "But we get all sorts of things. A bobcat last summer. And of course all kinds of white-tailed deer. And flying squirrels, red squirrels, gray squirrels."

"Flying squirrels? I thought you had to go to Borneo to see those."

"Well, they're similar. They have a little skin that joins their forelegs and hindlegs. They're fairly common. In fact, I've heard that they are as common as the gray squirrel, but people aren't aware of them because they are nocturnal and very secretive. They chatter a lot but their vocalizations are so high-pitched

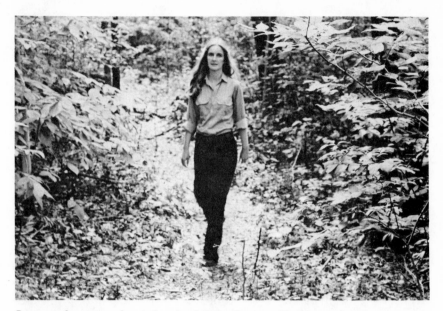

Jean on her rounds at the Audubon Center. To her trained eye, every step reveals minute details of a natural world largely hidden to uninitiated.

that you can walk through the woods at night and not even hear them."

I looked around hopefully, but no squirrels. My attention was caught by two trees only a few yards apart – one was young and thriving, the other withered.

"Red oak," said Jean, "and both the same age. We had a boring done on them, counted the rings."

The same age? How could that be? The first was fifteen feet around, the second a mere four or five feet.

Jean pointed to the healthy tree, which stood a few feet down the slope from its neighbor. "This one is in an area that drains naturally in the spring. There are pools here, so it gets plenty of water and the soil conditions are good. That one there is standing on rock. All the water runs off before it penetrates."

"Lucky to be alive at all, I suppose."

I looked around at the woodland again. What age was it? I wanted to know.

"Well, I would guess that this was allowed to grow back at about the turn of the century. We have some untouched areas toward the back of the property, but most of the other greenery

---

"Two roads diverged in a wood, and I –
I took the one less traveled by,
And that has made all the difference."

Robert Frost, "The Road Not Taken"

---

around here would be what I call 'teenage' growth. One day it's going to be mature oak-hickory in the upland areas and beech-maple-birch in some of the lowlands."

We stopped to examine some of the undergrowth. "Know what this is?" said Jean. "Spice bush." She picked a sprig. "Smell it. Just like a rather famous junk food. Can you think what it is?"

"It's familiar, but I can't place it."

"Seven-Up, of course. The scientific name for spice bush is *Lindera benzoin* because its leaves contain benzoic acid, an aromatic preservative. If you look at a Seven-Up can, you'll see benzoic acid listed in the ingredients."

We were now going downhill through the forest. Ahead, glimmering through the trees, lay Mead Lake. Water trickled over a spillway beside an old dam site, where at one time a saw mill had stood. I began to wonder if it was possible to establish an artificial environment like a lake and then leave it unmanaged.

"I reckon that long before the Meads arrived on the scene," Jean mused, "the only waterway that coursed through here was a branch of the river and they dammed it up to create the lake. It had been fairly stable until recently; but now we are having a problem with siltation. Largely due to management practices on the part of our neighbors."

I detected something in Jean's choice of words. "Meaning what?"

"Well, the way they have been using their land has caused a lot of runoff. There is one fellow in particular who likes to build ponds and move earth. He has his own bulldozers and essentially manipulates the land enough to loosen the earth, and it washes down into the lake."

So the ecology was changing. Would the sanctuary authorities let it change? Or would they intervene to keep it as it was? A philosophical problem for which Jean had no ready answer. Who could have?

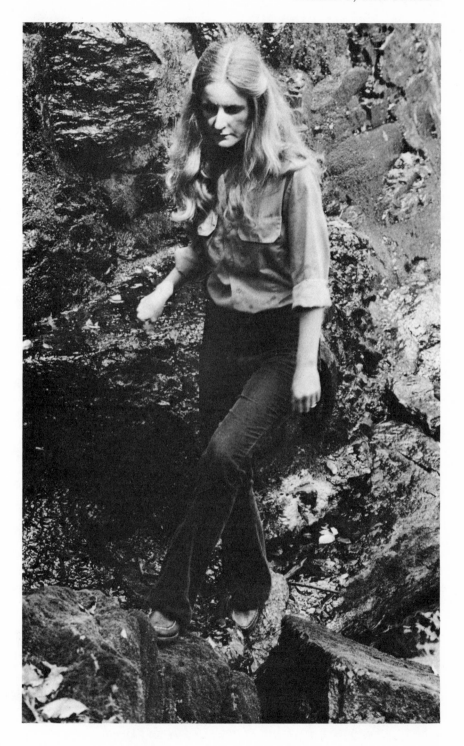

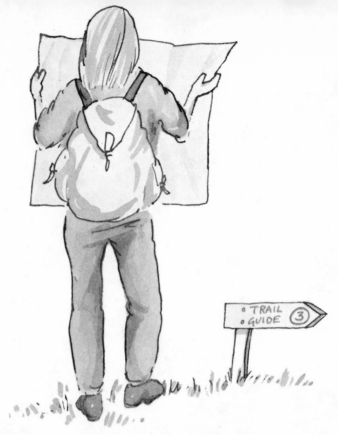

"We have perch and bass in there. We have even poled out American eels, fairly good-sized ones. We've had otter on the lake, ducks, Canada geese. The lake is an unbelievably rich habitat. We even have a carnivorous plant: bladderwort."

Bladderwort? It sounded revolting.

"Not at all," said Jean. "Look." We had arrived at the edge of the lake, and she pointed down at an innocuous-looking, seaweedy water plant. "It's fascinating stuff," she assured me. "It eats tiny little aquatic organisms like water fleas, which are no bigger than pinheads. It has bulbous growths all along it – little bladders – which work on a vacuum-and-trigger mechanism. If a little creature bumps into the bladder, a valve opens and the victim gets sucked in."

At every step as we made our way along the shore, Jean saw something that sparked a flood of comment – the moss on a rotting tree; an Oriental bittersweet vine winding parasitically around a tree; bloodroot, a member of the poppy family whose name is derived from the color of its sap (it was used as a dye by the Indians); a sensitive fern –

"Why sensitive?" I asked.

"Because it's one of the first green things to die in the cold of fall. And look at this little flower. It's a sort of arum, called Jack-in-the-Pulpit. See its flowers?"

I bent down. The flower was a cup, overhung with a lip-like leaf which hid the central stalk. "I suppose that's Jack," I said.

I stood up and suddenly noticed how quiet the woods were. "It's the time of day, plus the heat," she told me. "This is not prime time for birds to feed. They like dawn and dusk, and so do the mammals. That's when we'd see deer, raccoon, 'possum, river otter, although they don't inhabit any one area for great lengths of time. They tend to move on overland –"

"What was that?" I interrupted, responding to an odd noise nearby.

"An oven bird. It's a small warbler which spends most of its time on the ground; it even nests on the ground. It's named after its nest – a little bower of dried leaves that looks just like an old-fashioned earth oven."

"Is that its only call?"

"Yes, as far as I'm aware. At least around here."

"You mean in other parts of the country it might have other calls?"

"Sure. Birds have dialects like us. In other parts of the country, a bird of a certain species will often sound quite different. They tend to introduce little interesting twists to their commentary."

We came to the far end of the lake and turned along the boardwalk, which runs through an alder swamp with a host of saplings sticking up from the wet floor. Despite the swamp's designation, not all the saplings were alder; some were spice birch, some witch hazel, some red maple.

A gray dragonfly bobbed down at us, then flitted away. It occurred to me the swamp, like the man-made lake that formed it, would not last forever. "These lilies, now," I said, looking at the spreading pads that carpeted the water beyond the marsh, "they must look beautiful later on when the flowers come out. But don't they threaten to overwhelm the lake?"

"Well, their roots and their stalks trap and slow down the flow of water carrying the silt."

"What are you going to do about that? Dig it out?"

"We don't know how we're going to cope with it yet. One way would be to dredge it out, and it may come to that."

---

*"To learn something new, take the path today that you took
yesterday."*

John Burroughs

"Would you ever break the dam? Let the place revert to what
it was before the Meads arrived?"

"I doubt it. It's such a nice place, and we've just put in the
brand new boardwalk. Besides, it's not so unnatural. You
could compare damming like this to what beavers do. You can't
do more damage to the local ecology than beavers."

It was very hot out on the boardwalk. The air was muggy,
and the mosquitoes were beginning to nibble. We walked on
across the swamp, off the walkway and into the woods on the
other side. I realized a single visit here – or anywhere – was only
a beginning. I could come every day for ten years and see a
new world each time.

We were walking uphill now toward a dilapidated stone wall.
Suddenly a weasel poked its head out of a rocky niche in the
wall and transfixed us with a stare.

"What a thrill," said Jean, "I've only seen a couple of those
here before." She seemed about to thank the little creature in
person. We stood, the three of us, for a few long seconds until
the weasel broke the mood and scampered away along the wall,
a streak of red against gray.

"Wasn't that beautiful? He just stood there. Perhaps he'd
been relying on not being seen first and if we had continued
on our way without stopping and looking in his direction, he
probably would have stayed still until we were past.

"Did you notice that he was only about nine inches long?"
she went on. "A lot of people think they're bigger than they
are because they're such efficient predators."

"What do they find to eat here?"

"One of their well-known items of diet is the cotton-tail
rabbit. They bound after their prey, catapulting along with
their long backbones and in the last stride they leap in the air,
straddle the back of the prey and snap its neck with one bite.
The body plan of that little guy is an indication of how he gets
other meals. He is built like a tube, short and close to the
ground and narrow for going into burrows after a rabbit, for

example, or perhaps a meadow mouse, or a white-footed mouse. If he was hungry, I suppose he might also eat an occasional frog, or toad, or snake, but he prefers warm-blooded animals."

I had already learned in an afternoon more than I could ever have learned from books in a week. Moreover, I thought, I would remember it. We were walking down the other side of the lake now, past a bird blind. In the water near our feet, a sunfish was basking. Some fifteen feet from the shore, a snapping turtle broke the surface and then submerged. We walked onto a lakeside rock from which we could see into the middle of the lake.

"See the island?" Jean pointed out over the water. "We have a pair of Canada geese there. They return to the same base every spring. A lot of research is now being done on birds that mate for life. It looks as if they may not have an allegiance to each other, but an allegiance to a nest site."

We turned, continued along the lake, crossed the lower end over the dam, and headed back uphill through the woods toward the headquarters.

"That was beautiful," I said. "Does everybody who comes here think so?"

"Afterwards, yes. But sometimes, at first, people who are used to urban situations are a little bit worried about being lost."

"Even in this small area?"

"Yes. And concerned about what they will run into in the way of animal life. People tend to have exaggerated mental images of some of the predatory animals. If you ask some of the children that we get on school groups how big they think a fox is, they will describe something the size of a collie dog. When they leave, they know better. The fact is that this is a perfect place to start learning about nature. You can spend a few hours or a few years and get as much out of it as you want. You can use it as a wilderness in miniature or a large garden."

Well, I certainly got a lot out of the walk. After that, I promised myself that whenever I could I'd turn a walk into an education.

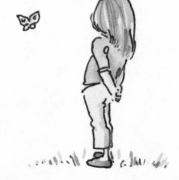

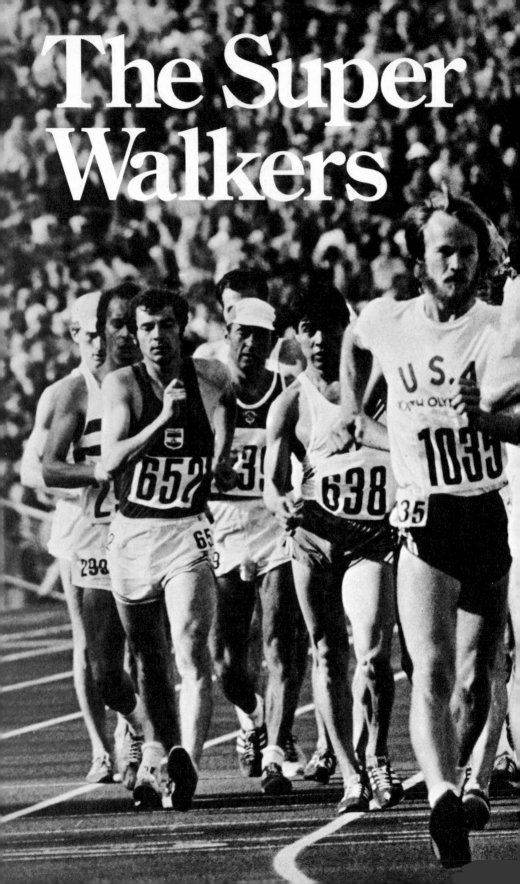

The Super Walkers

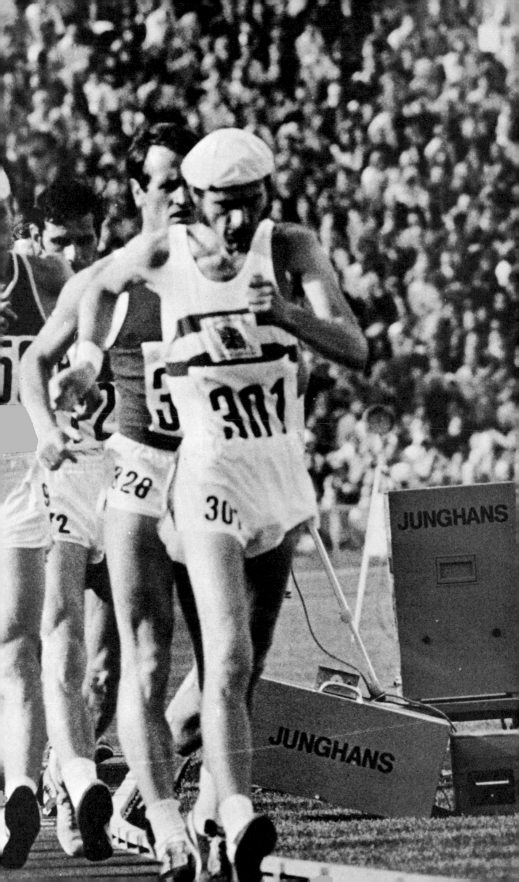

The Super Walkers

MOST OF THIS BOOK has been concerned with walking at a basic level for physical and emotional well-being. It has, in a way, been a foundation course in fitness. If you walk a few miles regularly, some of it uphill; if by walking you raise your heartbeat and can preserve your weight at a steady, healthy level, you are perfectly fit for normal life. Many people prefer to go on from there into any one of countless activities that seem to offer more of a challenge. If you're hooked on walking, though, and want to build onto that basic level of fitness that you've now achieved, why not go on and develop your walking abilities even further?

Walking itself can be among the most demanding of all physical activities. Some people specialize in speed – across the world there are thousands of race walkers (although it's an activity that has not, as yet, established a large following in the US.) Others concentrate on distance and speed. In England there is a club called the Centurions for people, only a few hundred at that, who have achieved the staggering feat of walking one hundred miles in twenty-four hours. And there are a few hearty souls who like to walk immense distances – around the coast of England, perhaps, or across the US – in the course of several weeks.

In all these activities there is an element of challenge, of competition. The walkers pit themselves against nature, against other walkers, against their own physical capacities. Historically, this is a fairly recent development. There have always been long-distance walkers, of course – like the Elizabethan eccentric, Tom Coryat, who walked across all Europe and finally headed for the Holy Land and on to India, where he died. There were medieval friars who would wander back and forth across Europe for the whole of their lives. But the idea of walking competitively really only took hold in the latter half of the eighteenth century, when the main interest of the sport was in gambling.

Peculiar, but Proud:
The Roots of Race Walking

Competitive pedestrianism reached its heyday in the second half of the nineteenth century, but eventually died away in the 1880s because there seemed no worthwhile records left to break; it was also becoming extremely hard to define the borderline between walking and running (a problem that still bedevils race walkers today).

The pedestrians usually raced against the clock rather than against other walkers. Events were held on main roads conveniently punctuated with milestones, or in parks, on race courses and across commons. Standard distances were adopted – 5, 10, 50 and 100 miles were the most usual – and onlookers placed bets for or against a particular distance being covered within a particular time, depending on the nature of the ground, the pedestrian's form and the weather. Occasionally a particularly bizarre attempt would arouse passionate public interest.

Some of the feats these super-pedestrians achieved now seem amazingly esoteric. One of the favorite standard events was to attempt to walk a given number of miles or part-miles in a successive number of hours or part-hours – 1,000 miles, say, in 1,000 successive hours – to test endurance: the walker could never sleep for more than a few minutes. When Richard Manks, for instance, achieved renown for walking 1,000 miles in 1,000 successive half-hours in 1851, he would walk a mile, then rest until the beginning of the next half-hour, then walk another mile; and so on. The combinations were never-ending. Walking wizard William Gale, for example, walked not only 1,500 miles in 1,000 successive hours, but on another occasion 4,000 quarter-miles in 4,000 successive quarter-hours.

Three men stand out as my real favorites in the peculiar story of pedestrians. First is Foster Powell, who was born in 1734 and made a minor reputation for himself as a young man by walking 50 miles in 7 hours – not a bad pace for a walker even today, and quite startling when one considers road conditions in the eighteenth century and the fact that Powell was encumbered with a great coat and leather breeches. In 1773 he walked from London to York and back again (402 miles) in 5 days 18 hours – an average of 72 miles a day. The feat made him something of a national hero. He left London at 12:20 AM on a Monday (November 29) and reached York at 2:00 PM on the Wednesday. He then slept for 1½ hours, started back at 5:30, and – sustained only by tea and toast – reached London again at 6:30 on Saturday evening. His return to town was heralded by a crowd of three thousand people on horseback and in carriages, who kept him company from Highgate. When he died, at the age of 59, a broadsheet mourned his passing:

> For quick ideas, some we praise,
> And men of talents meet;
> But this man's fame – and fame it was –
> Lay wholly in his Feet.
>
> Such Feet were never seen before;
> Witness this wond'rous work,
> (Which thousands long remember well)
> Of travelling to York.
>
> But now, alas! Poor Powell's gone
> To that mysterious bourn,
> From which the immortal Shakespeare says
> No trav'lers e'er return!

My second favorite, Captain Barclay (whose real name was Allardice: he preferred to keep an old family name) was immensely strong. At the age of 20, for a bet, he lifted half a ton (presumably on his shoulders; a tremendous feat, though the current world record for lifting a weight off trestles is over two tons). The Captain was also a stupendous walker. He once covered 40 miles to attend a dinner party. On one occasion he is said to have walked 30 miles while grouse shooting and then walked 60 miles home to attend to his business. In 1801 he undertook to walk 90 miles in 21½ hours, for 2,000 guineas, but brandy and nausea stopped him. He failed again and then, when a third attempt was suggested, this time with 5,000 guineas at stake, he decided to take the matter seriously. He trained remorselessly, once covering the whole 90 miles through heavy rain and often up to his ankles in mud. On the day of the event a mile was measured out on the York-Hull road; observers were stationed to notch the rounds on a turning post; lamps were placed; stop watches set; and Barclay accomplished the feat "strong and hearty," with 1 hour 8 minutes to spare.

He reached the pinnacle of his career when he became the first to walk 1,000 miles in 1,000 successive hours, a feat often attempted but never before achieved. Previous pedestrians had always succumbed to painfully swollen legs and feet or just plain exhaustion. A sum of £100,000 was wagered on the result – a staggering amount for those days. The match began at New-market at midnight on June 1, 1809, and lasted for 42 days, during which time Barclay had no more than half-hour snatches of sleep. He breakfasted at 5:00 AM on "roasted fowl, a pint of strong ale and two cups of tea, with bread and butter." At 12:00 he downed beef steaks and mutton chops on alternate days. He completed the course, 32 pounds lighter, at 3:00 PM on July 12 to the sound of church bells.

Third on my list is an extraordinary character named Edward Payson Weston – perhaps the most stupendous walker America has ever seen. His mother was a novelist and it is said that he developed a strong physique hawking her novels around Boston homes. In his youth he was, variously, a candy seller, jeweler and circus drummer (an occupation he abandoned after being struck by lightning, which he "took as a warning to quit that mode of life"). He later became a police reporter for the *New York Herald*, a job in which his ever-developing speed and endurance gave him a decided professional advantage.

Weston's first long-distance walk was from Boston to Washington, D.C., in 10 days – the idea being to arrive in the capital in time for Lincoln's inauguration. He made Washington, but missed the ceremony by a few hours. When he was 28, he walked the 1,326 miles from Portland, Maine, to Chicago, in 26 days – a time he would beat by 29 hours some forty years later, when he was 68.

In the 1870s Weston went to Britain, where he took part in a number of contests in London's Royal Agricultural Hall. In one, a 500-mile race, done as part of a six-day contest against Daniel O'Leary, another American, the contestants both put up £500. Before a crowd of twenty thousand, O'Leary won in 5 days 14 hours, with a commanding lead of 22 miles. Both went

AGRICULTURAL HALL,

ISLINGTON.

EASTER MONDAY

AND FIVE FOLLOWING DAYS.

April 2nd 1877

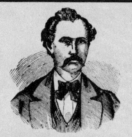

DANIEL O'LEARY.

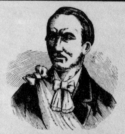

EDWARD PAYSON WESTON.

O'LEARY v. WESTON

FOR

£1000

These celebrated Long Distance Walkers will Meet for the First Time in England, and Contest in a Fair and Legitimate Manner for

The Largest Amount of Money ever Walked for in the World!!

The whole of which has been Deposited in the hands of "Sporting Life."
Each Man will Walk upon a Separate Track.—Five Judges from the principal London Newspapers have been Appointed

TWO MILITARY BANDS.

ADMISSION—One Shilling.

Matthews Brothers, Printers, Thomas Street, Paradise Street, Liverpool.

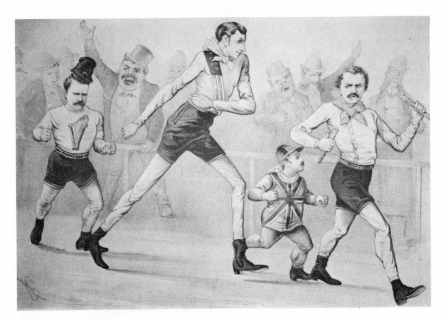

"The Great Walk – Go as You Please": an 1879 lithograph by Thomas Worth, evoking the passions aroused by the international pedestrian races of the late nineteenth century.

on to complete the six days, covering 520 and 510 miles respectively.

Then, in 1879, Weston agreed to attempt a 2,000-mile tour in 1,000 hours, undertaking at the same time to give fifty lectures about his walking experiences along the way. He did it for a bet of £500, against his own £100, laid by a certain Sir John Astley, who stipulated that Weston should not walk on Sundays – but that the time spent thus in rest should be deducted from the total time available, leaving him only 856 hours. Undaunted, Weston set off from the Royal Exchange in London on January 8 and headed along terrible roads through a snowstorm to Folkestone, $81\frac{1}{2}$ miles away. Toward the end of the tour, he was left with 31 hours to cover 105 miles back into London, an easy enough feat in normal circumstances, but with twelve hours to go, he fell asleep and lost three hours. At 4:00 PM, when his time was up, he still had $22\frac{1}{2}$ miles to go. A sport to the end, he finished anyway, £100 poorer.

In 1909, at the age of 70, Weston walked from New York to San Francisco in 104 days 7 hours – an average of 37 miles a day. The following year he walked the return journey – though by a shorter route – in 77 days. At the age of 88, while out walking, he was struck by a taxi and crippled. He died two years later.

I have two other small anecdotes about pedestrians. First concerns an Englishman named George Wilson, who gamely tried to walk 1,000 miles in 20 days over a one-mile course at Blackheath in 1815. Wilson was "by no means well made," according to a contemporary pen portrait. "His shoulders are rather broad, but his arms are disproportionately long; his legs and thighs are awkwardly hung together." Unfortunately, it was the even longer arm of the law that prevented Wilson from attaining his goal: after covering 750 miles, he was arrested (rather unfairly, it seems to me) for causing an undue crush of people on the heath.

And finally, there is James Hocking of Teaneck, New Jersey, who, in 1924, at the age of 68, walked from Coney Island to San Francisco in 75 days, averaging 50 miles a day. The international Mark Twain Society recognized Hocking's "outstanding contributions to American sport" by electing him to honorary membership of the society on his ninety-sixth birthday in October 1952. He died in 1954 at the age of 98, having covered an estimated 270,000 miles in his lifetime.

A Rare Breed:
The Super-Distance Walkers

The indirect descendants of nineteenth-century pedestrianism are hard, long walks in all their forms, whether on a track, along roads or over the countryside. So far these are a peculiarly European phenomenon (although the Mexicans are up-and-coming race walkers). Americans may take to the trails for days at a time, but there is as yet little tradition of 20-kilometer and 50-kilometer walking (the two Olympic race-walking events); and there seems to be little of the competitive drive that compels English people to undertake "challenge walks," as they are known, of anything up to 100 miles. There is no US equivalent, for example, to the Long-Distance Walkers Association which has two thousand members. The association sponsors walks the very names of which sound formidable – the Downsman 100, the Fellsman Hike, The Tanner's Marathon, Six Shropshire Summits.

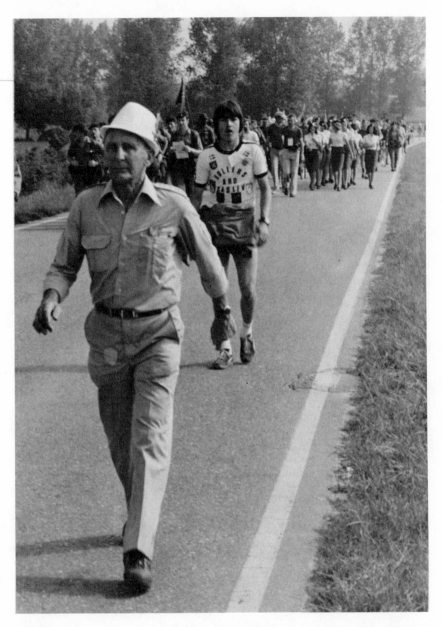

A nation of walkers: some of the 17,500 participants in the annual four-day walking event at Nijmegen, Holland. Walkers must cover 30 to 50 kilometers per day, depending on their age and sex. The walk – which attracts entrants from thirty nations – has been held since 1909, and has inspired similar events throughout the Netherlands (which has over 500,000 "event" walkers) and most other European nations.

217

Why do they do it? Chris Steer, editor of the Long-Distance Walkers' journal *Strider* told me: "It's a combination of sheer joy and sheer hell. A long cross-country walk is a poor man's Everest. You have to find your own way across the wildest country, and do it in a set time – 24 or 36 hours. But it's not too expensive. We don't camp. And we have the best system of footpaths in the world and the best maps to go by. Then, of course, there's the sense of achievement – imagine the Fellsman Walk in West Yorkshire: 59 miles over several 2,000-foot peaks in 24 hours! Or the Bob Graham Round – named after the chap who was the first to do it – 75 miles over 42 Lake District summits! We're a rare breed, but we're growing all the time."

Perhaps the most esoteric club of all is that of the Centurions, those people who have covered 100 miles in 24 hours. Amazingly, this achievement has an increasing appeal. Each year the LDWA organizes a 100-mile cross-country walk somewhere in England, and although the event is never a race and there are no prizes to be won, so many people wish to take up the challenge that the entry list has to be restricted to 250. The Centurions, until recently an all-male preserve, changed their rules in 1977 to allow women members. They did so to accommodate Ann Sayer, 41, who had already completed an unofficial 100 miles in 24 hours in the Netherlands. At Bristol in 1977 she completed her 100 miles in 20 hours 37 minutes. In a field of 82, only 56 of whom finished, Ann placed eleventh, to qualify as Centurion Number 599.

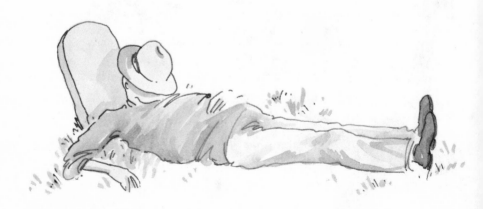

The Hip Swivelers

The other type of competitive walking is race walking, with its hip-swiveling action that can propel a good walker along at a spanking 9 MPH or more. To my mind, race walking combines two great advantages for those who like doing it: it is extremely demanding, yet it is also almost totally injury free.

Race walking was first included in the Olympics in 1908. This marked the beginning of a slow but steady renaissance of the sport as competitors and officials worked toward a satisfactory definition of race walking. The official definition now reads as follows:

Walking is progression by steps, so taken that unbroken contact with the ground is maintained. . . . During the period of each step when a foot is on the ground, the leg must be straightened (i.e., not bent at the knee) at least for one moment, and, in particular, the supporting leg must be straight in the vertical upright position.

These are hard rules to follow when walking at running speed, and in international races hawk-eyed judges hover alongside the track ready with warnings (two are allowed) and disqualifications.

The technique itself is surprisingly demanding. As the leading foot makes contact with the ground, it decelerates the body. The walker has to pull the heel backwards and drive hard with his rear leg, to carry himself over the top of the leading foot. At the same time he has to swing his hips to gain the extra 6 to 8 inches that the width of the pelvis confers.

Arm drive, too, is vital. The arm swing does two things. Firstly, the swing of the arms round the body counteracts the eccentricity imposed by the rotating hip movement. Secondly, as one arm swings forward and the other backward, both simultaneously swing upward. There is an equal and opposite reaction downward, increasing pressure on the ground through the supporting leg. This, in its turn, enables the walker to propel himself forward at a faster rate.

The physical benefits of race walking are akin to running. Good walkers have startling endurance. Walking at speed strengthens all the leg muscles, the flexor muscles of the hip, the stomach muscles and the muscles in the lower back. In

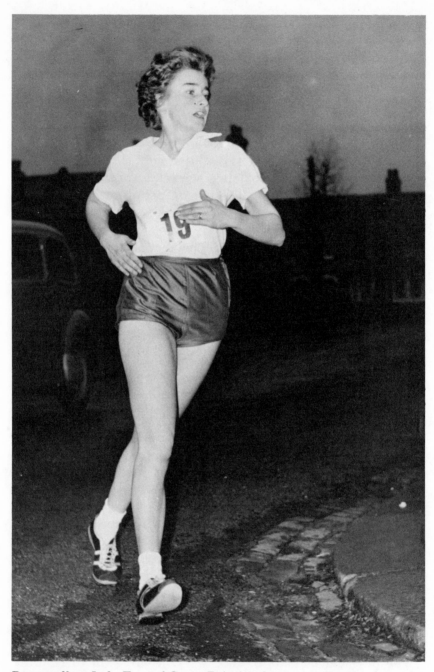

Race walker Judy Farr of Great Britain, demonstrating the dynamic leg and arm action that requires so much concentration and fitness.

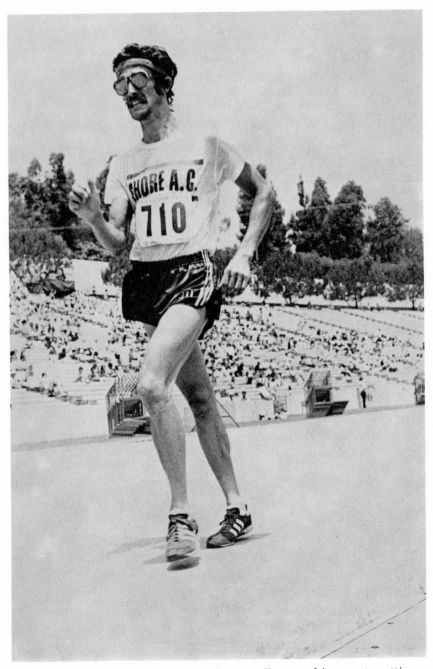

Todd Scully, champion American race walker, on his way to setting a meet record in the 20 kilometer event of the 1978 National AAU Outdoor Track and Field Championships at UCLA's Drake Stadium.

THE FURTHEST AND THE FASTEST

Probably the longest and toughest walk ever undertaken in modern times was that made by Sebastian Snow who in nineteen months walked from the southernmost point of South America to Panama, a distance of nearly 9,000 miles.

The transcontinental Los Angeles-to-New York record (2,876 miles) was set in 1972 by Englishman John Lees with a time of 53 days and $12\frac{1}{4}$ hours.

One record that has stood the test of time is the 7 hours 35 minutes for the $52\frac{1}{2}$ miles London-to-Brighton road walk, set by Don Thompson in 1957.

The longest mass walk in England was probably the Lands End-to-John O'Groats walk of 1960. Organized by Butlins, over three thousand would-be marathon walkers aimed to cover the nearly 900-mile trek from the northeast of Scotland to the southwest of England. Only 113 men and 25 women reached the finish, with J. Musgrave the first home in 15 days and 14 hours.

Here is a check list of some other records:

Official Records (Track)

Event	Time (or Distance)	Record Breaker	Date
20km	1hr 23mins 31.9secs	Daniel Bautista (Mex.)	May 14, 1977
30km	2hrs 11mins 53.4secs	Raul Gonzalez (Mex.)	May 19, 1978
50km	3hrs 52mins 23.5secs	Raul Gonzalez (Mex.)	May 19, 1978
2hrs	27km 247m	Raul Gonzalez (Mex.)	May 19, 1978

Unofficial Records (Track)

Event	Time (or Distance)	Record Breaker	Date
1mile	5mins 53.2secs (i)	Reima Salonen (Fin.)	Feb. 2, 1977
3km	11mins 5.1secs (i)	Reima Salonen (Fin.)	Feb. 2, 1977
5km	19mins 26.2secs	Karl-Heinz Stadtmuller (GDR)	June 22, 1975
10km	39mins 39.9secs	Daniel Bautista (Mex.)	June 2, 1978
100km	9hrs 23mins 58.6secs	Roger Quemener (Fr.)	Mar. 28, 1976
100mi	17hrs 18mins 51.0secs	Hugh Neilson (GB)	Oct. 15, 1960
1hr	14km 430m	Daniel Bautista (Mex.)	May 28, 1978
24hr	219km 500m	Derek Harrison (GB)	May 20, 1978

Unofficial Records (Road)

Event	Time (or Distance)	Record Breaker	Date
20km	1hr 23mins 11.5secs	Roland Weiser (GDR)	Aug. 8, 1978
50km	3hrs 41mins 19.2secs	Raul Gonzalez	June 11, 1978
100km	9hrs 15mins 57.4secs	Christoph Hohne (GDR)	Oct. 29, 1967
20mi	2hrs 22mins 53.0secs	Daniel Bautista (Mex.)	May 22, 1976

(i) = indoor performance

addition, walking demands a considerable mobility in the shoulders, trunk, hips and ankles.

Newcomers should take heed: the demands are very different from running. If you've never done it before, a quarter mile in $2\frac{1}{2}$ minutes (6 MPH) is agony, especially for the muscles along the shin.

So, race walking is tough and good for you; but how much joy is there in it? To answer this question, I spoke to Paul Nihill, former world record holder at 20 kilometers, European champion and four-time Olympic competitor. Nihill began as a runner but broke his knee when he was 20 and took up walking after that. Within three years he'd reached national standard and decided to press on seriously. He competed in his first Olympics in 1964 and, despite retiring a number of times, he has always come back. Has he retired now? "I'm not sure. Perhaps I'll go for my fifth Olympics."

Nihill's training schedule was grueling. When he was at the top, he did three hours a day and five on Sundays. He combined this with speed work – half-miles at $9\frac{1}{2}$ MPH; miles in just over six minutes each. It was workouts like this over the years that enabled him to walk 20 kilometers at about $8\frac{1}{2}$ MPH. He claims the sport is far more demanding than running. "It takes in-

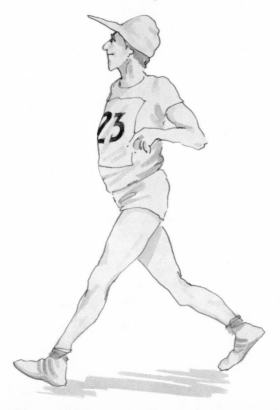

credible concentration. You can never relax. In running, you can run like hell, but in walking you have to concentrate all the time on *not* running."

His career has taken its toll. "I was always a reluctant walker," he said, "and walking is very much a Cinderella sport. I got terrific satisfaction from traveling around as a top competitor and from winning. And I've always enjoyed the comradeship. Walkers are a cliquish lot and it's good to face a common challenge." But after a time, the sport palled for him. He speaks now as if he's had all the walking burned out of him. "I'm more of a recluse now. I never watch walking races. I feel it's a bit like a job: when you retire, you don't want anything more to do with it. Now I can enjoy a good run without someone saying, 'Hey, you're running.' It's more fun and I move faster."

Surely that's just a personal reaction? "No, it's not just me. A number of top walkers – like Ken Matthews and Stan Vickers – have also pulled out of the sport."

That sounded depressing. I asked Britain's national coach in walking events, Julian Hopkins, about the problem. He was reassuring. The light and stringy Hopkins, who trains more than 60 miles a week, has never been bored by the sport, perhaps because he has the natural build of a walker. "I haven't got the muscle power for sprinting," he says.

For him, it is precisely the technical demands of the sport that preserve the interest. He finds that the restrictions demand determination and will power. Moreover, he takes joy in the pure mechanical efficiency of the activity. "I'm always looking for a feeling of flowing along – the equivalent of a running 'high.' It's beautiful to achieve.

"Injuries? The only trouble I've ever had is with the muscles in the front of the shin. If you think about it, these muscles, which hold up the front of the foot, never get much rest in walking. I never heard of anyone developing Achilles tendon or hamstring trouble, which runners get. And race walking eliminates the rise and fall of the trunk. You don't have to lift a great weight as you do in running, so walking allows people of different builds to compete fairly equally.

"Boredom may be a problem for some people, but remember that race-walking careers are far longer than those of runners. It's an activity that's suitable for all ages. There are many internationals in their early 40s, and you can compete at a

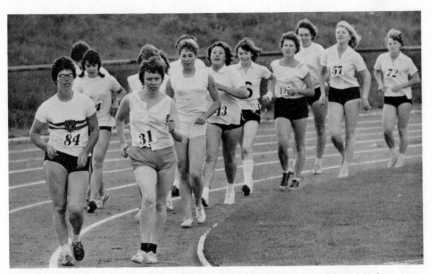

Women's race walking, though popular enough to sustain regular events like this one at Hayes, Middlesex, in Britain, is not recognized officially. A number of women walkers are campaigning for recognition by the 1984 Olympics. This event featured the international pentathalete Mary Rand (without number), *who finished fifth.*

high level until you're 50, almost on a par with 20-year-olds."

Certainly, achievement must be the great spur, and the sport – largely because it is now permanently in the Olympics – is growing internationally. The English have lost their world lead to the East Germans, Russians and Mexicans, where full-time, state-supported walkers have achieved unparalleled performances. Mexico's Daniel Bautista, has walked over 8 miles in the space of one hour. Reima Salonen of Finland has walked a mile in 5 minutes 53 seconds – a fraction over 10 MPH.

In the United States the sport has not yet come alive. Elliott Denman, one of the keenest of America's walkers, told me that there are only about a thousand people involved in the sport. But he swears its popularity is growing. Like Julian Hopkins, he has never had any problem with boredom. "From the time I was a teenager, I walked for the sake of walking," he said. "Walking is the greatest activity going. It only *looks* boring, but I find it terrific to test myself and terrific to meet new people. Joggers talk about getting 'highs,' but I get all the highs they get. Over in England, I walked from London to Brighton, and it was a magnificent feeling. . . ."

The Loneliness of the Long-Distance Walker

And what of those who go really long distances? What do they get out of walking? Take John Merrill, 34, who on November 8, 1978, completed one of the longest walks ever – 7,000 miles around the coast of England in ten months. He set out on January 3 carrying fifty pounds of equipment. Averaging 24 miles a day, he tramped through storms and was almost blown off clifftops. In Wales he diverted inland to climb Mount Snowdon – the first time he'd been out of earshot of the sea for 3 months – and he actually found himself in tears as he turned his back to the sea. At the Scottish border he developed a fatigue fracture of the toe and spent two weeks recovering, then climbed a few local peaks to get back into shape. From his journey he derived a sense of freedom and satisfaction from the knowledge that he was driving himself to the limits of physical and mental endurance. "It was the most marvelous sense of remoteness to be alone in that wonderful dramatic country."

Achievement, companionship, fitness – yes. But what else? For an answer I went to see John Hillaby, the acknowledged master-walker of Britain, who talked with characteristic passion about his life and his walking. He is a lean, white-haired 61-year-old, with enough experience of the world for a man twice his age and the exuberance of a teenager. Newspaperman, writer, natural historian, Hillaby began his professional walking-writing career with a journey from Wamba in North Kenya to Lake Rudolf and back, a distance of 1,100 miles.

"I calculate that with these identical legs W. (Wordsworth) must have traversed a distance of 175,000 to 180,000 English miles – a mode of exertion which, to him, stood in the stead of alcohol and all other stimulants."

Christopher Morley, *The Art of Walking*

"When a traveller asked Wordsworth's servant to show him her master's study, she answered, 'Here is his library, but his study is out of doors.' . . ."

Henry David Thoreau, *Walking*

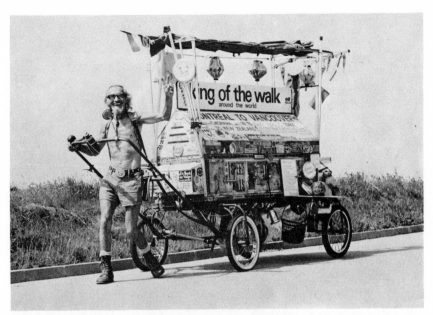

Foot-slogging caravaner Elzear Duquette, a French-Canadian, has walked across Europe and much of Asia. Here he is in his sixties in 1972, heading for Munich to watch the Olympics.

"As a correspondent, I got heartily fed up whizzing into various cities in Europe and Africa without ever seeing anything of the places. Eventually, I thought, 'My God, what am I missing?' After a conference in Arusha, in what I still call Tanganyika, I went on a series of post-conference tours. One of them led me into North Kenya, where, with a game warden, I went up into the highlands. This particular game warden, who was a pretty rough character, said 'From here, on a good day, you can see Lake Rudolf. That is a remarkable place,' and he pointed to what must have represented about one hundred miles of bloody awful terrain. I said, 'How do you get there?' He said, 'You walk!'

"That started me. My personal life was in a bit of a mess, and it seemed a good time to get away. I did a lot of homework, mind you. I learned Swahili. I learned to shoot. And then I had just over three months' walking. It was exhilarating. Something was *happening* – not every day, but every hour. I hadn't been there two days before I'd forgotten what it was I'd come to forget. So I thought, well, this is marvelous. I suddenly realized what a wonderful world it was to walk in."

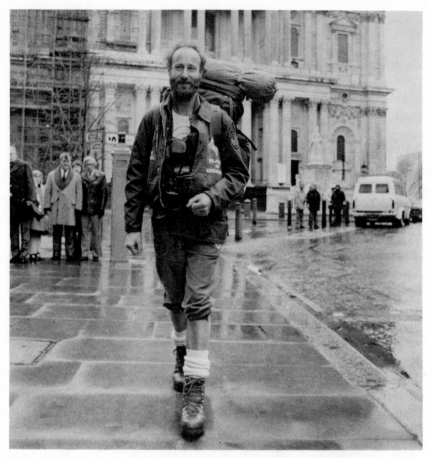

John Merrill, setting out from St. Paul's, London, on January 3,
1978, at the beginning of his 7,000-mile walk around the coasts of
Britain.

Since then he's walked from Land's End to John o'Groats
and from the Hook of Holland to Nice. His books on these great
walks are marvelous patchworks of incident, anecdote, myth-
ology, history and commentary. People, customs and natural
history combine to reveal a passion for life that is both physical
and intellectual – the very spirit of walking.

I asked him whether he could see any sense in walking far or
fast just for the sake of it. He couldn't.

"My longest walk, for instance, was from here in this very
room in Hampstead, during a time of my life when I was un-
happily married. I decided to pop down to the pub to have a
drink with the boys. I got there about 7:00 PM. I found the two

biggest bores I knew, apart from myself, and thought 'Well, to hell with it.' So I walked down to my favorite drinking club in Piccadilly. It took me 1 hour 20 minutes. There I found three more bores and thought I'd move on again.

"I was rather depressed and remembered an old army chum of mine – a 'b. & e.' boy – breaking and entering, you know, a burglar. He's straight now and runs a nice pub in the Old Kent Road. I decided to walk down there. I must have got to the Old Kent Road about quarter past nine. He wasn't in so I thought 'To hell with it, I know a chap in Purley.' So I went on there. I'm not quite sure when I got to Purley, but when I got there, I decided I might as well go on to Brighton. I went on – Horley, Haywards Heath – on and on. Anyhow, to cut a tedious story short, I got to Brighton about quarter to eleven the following morning – 63 miles. That's probably about the longest walk I've ever done. And, God, was I bored! Never again!

"For a good deal of the time – and I suspect that most walkers would feel this – you tend to think 'What am I doing? If you walk as I do, for anything up to $2\frac{1}{2}$ months, you're very conscious that a lot of the time there's nothing particularly interesting happening to you and there's nothing to do but fall back on one's own mental resources" – in his case, a love of geology, natural history and history.

For John Hillaby, it's a love that is inbred. "I was born and lived my early years in Leeds, in Yorkshire. I can't pretend even now that I knew what I wanted to be, but I sought to make the best I could from local circumstances. Without realizing it, I began walking. My primary driving interest in those days was fly fishing. I used to go to the Dales in Yorkshire, and if the fishing wasn't up to scratch I'd think nothing of going over the top and dropping down into the next valley, which might mean a walk of anything up to twelve miles. Like our local flock masters – sheep farmers to you – I developed a fine gait.

"I was very fortunate. Living in Leeds was marvelous for me, because, although I had no university training I became passionately interested – without knowing it at the time – in natural history. In the 1930s Leeds University was living through a golden age. As a teenager I kept company with geologists, botanists and ecologists of all kinds (though the word was not used then). I was brought up to believe that most people are interested in what they see around them. I often went for walks in the country at weekends or on days off from school with people who could put a name to almost everything they saw – bird, plant, rock, mineral or whatever. As a child, I thought this was the norm. I assumed that if you went for a walk you should not only be able to say that such-and-such a flower was a buttercup, but which species of buttercup it was (there are eight, you know). It took me many years to realize that this was a peculiarity.

"I now realize that the norm is very different. It's dominated by what I call the Funicular Effect. I've walked several times through various bits of France and Switzerland, where mountain railways are common. Well, you get to the top of these damn funiculars; everybody bundles out; they all look round; they see a fantastic vista, Alps, peak upon peak, marching into the distance; they all go 'Ooh, aah, *c'est magnifique, wunderbar.*' Then everybody gets cold and they all trickle back to have coffee and dreadful green things in glasses and take photographs of each other. It's quite obvious, if you stand among them, that the average mind's capacity for interest before a great vista is two minutes at the most. It's not surprising. It's very difficult to look at anything for very long unless you understand something about it. This is where I've been lucky. I know something of what I experience, and that's what sustains me.

"Mental preoccupation is terribly important. Let me try and extend that a little. Fundamentally, I'm a newspaper man. I like to joke that I've been on three local papers, the *Dewsbury District News,* the *Manchester Guardian* and the *New York Times.* I was a science correspondent, which meant I had to pretend to a sort of polymathic ability, often on subjects I knew relatively little about. But I've picked up a bit over the years. Before I set off on a major walk, I spend up to six months reading and looking at maps. I have to have some preknowledge, as it were, of what I'm walking through. I know that when I pass such-and-such a place on my route, I shall be switching from sedimentary rock – say carboniferous limestone – to granite. As I walk, I try to answer questions. Is there any immediate change in the appearance of the land? Is it more rugged because it's harder to erode? Can I notice the effects in plants which are specific to a particular geology? These are the sort of things that keep me going.

"But then, of course, I don't go on forever. In my walks of

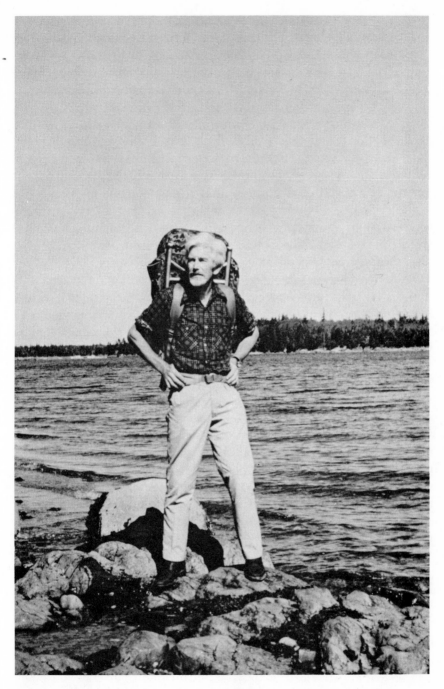

Britain's long-distance walker John Hillaby on the banks of the Penobscot River in Maine.

"Tramping is a way of approach, to Nature, to your fellow man, to a nation, to a foreign nation, to beauty, to life itself."

Stephen Graham: *The Gentle Art of Tramping*

---

over 1,000 miles, I find that something cracks, something breaks about every 200 miles, and I find that I get psychologically tired. It's happened too often to be chance. Somewhere between 180 and 220 miles, a feeling comes over me that something's wrong. It's a sort of tiredness, as if the whole business of path-finding, of not knowing quite where you are, is too much. I have to relax, to stop and do something different. I break the walk for two or three days and occupy myself with something else. I talk, I eat, I read.

"If I don't know an area I usually find someone to tell me about it. If I suddenly came before God tomorrow morning and he asked what I really knew about, I think I might be tempted to say that I'm an expert in experts. One of the happiest walks I had was from the North Sea to the Mediterranean, which was a matter of about 1,300 miles. In each place I met somebody who knew a lot about the area. In Holland my mentor was a school mistress, Annie. She knew most about painting and she was able to describe the Dutch and their landscape. At Valkens-waard I met the chief falconer of Holland, who explained to me why the kings of Europe used to get all their birds from the place which is embodied in the town's name (it's directly on the great falcon migration route). There were many others. Though they were usually with me only for a short time – I don't like company much on the whole – I was extraordinarily grateful to these people. Through them and my own knowledge I lived the landscapes I walked through."

As he talked, I saw through his words the essence of walking. Walking means seeing the unseen, understanding, friendship, privacy, emotional perspective, physical capacity. A large claim, perhaps, for such a natural activity? Not really, because walking is, in the end, and image of life itself.

The Walker's Yellow Pages

Appendix 1
How to assess your own chances of developing heart disease

This table will enable you to assess your risk of heart disease, assuming you have access to medical information derived from a standard medical checkup. It is a more sophisticated version of the table on p. 62.

RISK FACTOR	RELATIVE LEVEL OF RISK				
	VERY LOW	LOW	MODER-ATE	HIGH	VERY HIGH
Blood pressure (mmHg)					
Systolic	<110	120	130–140	150–160	170+
Diastolic	< 70	76	82–88	94–100	105+
Cigarettes (per day)	Never	5	10–20	30–40	50+
Cholesterol (mm/100 cc)	<180	200	220–240	260–280	300+
Triglycerides (mm/100 cc)	< 80	100	150	200	300+
Glucose (mg/100 cc)	< 80	90	100–110	120–130	140+
Body fat (%) – Men	< 12	16	22	25	30+
Women	< 15	20	25	33	40+
Stress-Tension	Almost never	Occasional	Frequent	Nearly constant	
Physical endurance: weekly activity above a rate of 6 calories per minute (walking speed, about 4 mph)	4 hrs.	2–3 hrs.	$1\frac{1}{2}$–3 hrs.	$\frac{1}{2}$–1 hr.	Under $\frac{1}{2}$ hr.
Family history of premature heart attack* (blood relative)	0	1	2	3	4+
Age	< 30	35	40	50	60+

* Premature heart attack – i.e., under 60 years of age.

Appendix 2

Physical Fitness and Health Standards

These tables show how a number of medical factors range across the medical spectrum of an average Western population. When seeing where you fit in, remember that "average" does not mean "ideal."

You can assess your "Percentile Rankings" as follows:

Above 90	High
70–90	Above Average
40–69	Average
20–39	Below Average
Under 20	Low

	PERCENTILE RANKINGS	RESTING HEART RATE (beats/min)	RESTING BLOOD PRESSURE		MAXIMUM HEART RATE (beats/min)	CHOLES- TEROL (mg%)	FAT (%)
			SYSTOLIC (mmHg)	DIASTOLIC (mmHg)			
MEN AGED 20-29	99	40	94	60	214	120	7.2
	90	50	110	70	205	154	11.6
	80	54	112	72	200	165	13.9
	70	58	118	78	199	178	16.2
	60	60	120	80	197	190	18.0
	50	63	121	80	194	199	20.1
	40	66	128	80	191	207	22.3
	30	70	130	84	188	218	25.4
	20	72	136	88	183	229	28.6
	10	80	140	90	179	251	32.8
MEN AGED 30-39	99	40	96	60	210	135	7.1
	90	50	108	70	200	169	13.4
	80	55	110	74	198	182	16.2
	70	58	116	78	194	193	18.2
	60	60	120	80	191	203	20.1
	50	63	120	80	189	215	22.0
	40	65	124	81	186	224	23.6
	30	68	130	85	183	235	25.5
	20	72	132	90	180	250	28.0
	10	77	140	92	174	271	32.2

| | PERCENTILE RANKINGS | RESTING HEART RATE (beats/min) | RESTING BLOOD PRESSURE | | MAXIMUM HEART RATE (beats/min) | CHOLES- TEROL (mg%) | FAT (%) |
			SYSTOLIC (mmHg)	DIASTOLIC (mmHg)			
MEN AGED 40-49	99	42	96	60	205	145	9.2
	90	50	110	70	196	175	14.9
	80	54	111	76	191	193	17.7
	70	58	118	80	188	204	19.7
	60	60	120	80	185	214	21.5
	50	62	121	80	182	225	23.0
	40	65	126	84	180	235	24.6
	30	69	130	88	176	245	26.3
	20	72	138	90	171	257	28.5
	10	78	142	98	164	275	32.2
MEN AGED 50-59	99	42	98	60	200	149	9.0
	90	50	110	72	188	185	15.8
	80	55	116	78	183	201	18.4
	70	58	120	80	180	211	20.4
	60	60	122	80	176	220	22.1
	50	63	128	82	173	230	23.8
	40	65	130	86	170	240	25.4
	30	68	138	90	166	250	27.0
	20	72	140	90	160	264	29.1
	10	77	150	100	150	285	32.8
MEN AGED 60 AND OVER	99	38	98	60	195	152	10.5
	90	52	112	70	184	180	14.1
	80	55	120	76	175	196	17.2
	70	58	124	80	170	205	18.9
	60	60	130	80	165	214	20.8
	50	62	131	81	162	225	22.3
	40	65	140	84	159	234	24.4
	30	68	140	88	152	250	26.9
	20	72	150	90	145	264	28.9
	10	77	160	98	131	280	32.5

	PERCENTILE RANKINGS	RESTING HEART RATE (beats/min)	RESTING BLOOD PRESSURE SYSTOLIC (mmHg)	DIASTOLIC (mmHg)	MAXIMUM HEART RATE (beats/min)	CHOLES-TEROL (mg%)	FAT (%)
WOMEN AGED 20-29	99	48	90	56	213	135	4.8
	90	55	100	63	203	150	11.6
	80	59	101	68	198	165	15.1
	70	60	106	70	194	170	18.3
	60	63	110	72	190	182	23.2
	50	65	112	75	188	190	24.9
	40	70	118	78	186	196	26.2
	30	72	120	80	182	210	28.2
	20	75	120	80	180	219	33.3
	10	84	130	82	172	251	38.5
FEMALES AGED 30-39	99	48	90	60	210	124	5.1
	90	55	100	65	196	158	13.1
	80	58	104	70	192	168	16.7
	70	62	110	70	189	176	19.3
	60	65	110	74	185	188	21.5
	50	68	114	76	184	195	23.6
	40	70	118	80	182	204	25.5
	30	74	120	80	180	211	27.6
	20	76	122	82	176	224	31.3
	10	82	130	90	170	240	38.1
FEMALES AGED 40-49	99	43	90	58	208	130	7.3
	90	55	100	65	192	171	15.8
	80	60	105	70	186	184	19.6
	70	62	110	70	183	195	21.9
	60	64	112	75	180	201	23.9
	50	66	118	80	177	210	25.9
	40	70	120	80	173	217	27.6
	30	72	120	80	170	228	29.1
	20	76	130	82	166	241	31.4
	10	80	138	90	158	264	37.4

236

| | PERCENTILE RANKINGS | RESTING HEART RATE (beats/min) | RESTING BLOOD PRESSURE | | MAXIMUM HEART RATE (beats/min) | CHOLES- TEROL (mg%) | FAT (%) |
			SYSTOLIC (mmHg)	DIASTOLIC (mmHg)			
FEMALES AGED 50-59	99	45	90	58	202	158	10.8
	90	55	108	69	185	180	18.2
	80	60	110	70	180	198	22.7
	70	61	118	75	176	205	25.1
	60	64	120	79	173	218	27.0
	50	67	122	80	170	225	28.4
	40	69	130	82	167	234	30.4
	30	72	134	85	162	241	32.5
	20	75	140	90	160	260	34.7
	10	83	148	92	152	275	39.7
FEMALES AGED 60 AND OVER	98	46	110	66	178	127	6.8
	90	52	120	70	176	185	17.7
	80	57	120	75	165	210	22.2
	70	60	125	76	160	223	25.1
	60	62	128	80	155	235	27.1
	50	64	130	80	153	240	29.8
	40	66	136	80	150	245	30.8
	30	72	140	84	145	262	31.7
	20	74	142	88	140	269	34.7
	10	79	160	98	126	276	36.3

Data comes from the Cooper Clinic Coronary Risk Factor Profile Charts. Reproduced with permission.

Appendix 3
A Basic Walking Program

This program should be read and followed in conjunction with Chapter 4, "Step by Step." Before beginning the program, you must determine your fitness category, which can be done with the aid of the table opposite.

First take your resting heartbeat, and then work out your training heartbeat as described on pp. 93–4. Next do some experiments on a flat surface out of doors to discover which of the five fitness categories you fall into (Category 1 is the least fit; Category 5 is well above average). Only you can decide which level to start at, and you may have to walk two or three quarter-miles (440 yards) to find out. Don't push yourself: if you feel tired, slow down. Your heartbeat is not the only criteria. Your muscles have to adapt as well, so start in the fitness category that is well within your capacity.

The six-month program that follows for each of the five fitness categories is approximate. Paces per minute are included to help you establish a rhythm; they are not intended to tie you in to a rigid system. The "Total Time" column is also approximate, as are the "Calories Expended" (which have been calculated on an individual of 154 pounds, or 70 kilos).

As in running, the secret of building fitness is to build speed and endurance. The program outlined for Fitness Category 1 and most of Fitness Category 2 concentrates on developing endurance. It allows several months for the body to build the necessary muscular strength to cope with the demands people normally place on their bodies. Beyond this foundation fitness, which is organized in terms of a steady increase in mileage, the programs suggest an alternation of shorter distances and paces, which allows a gradual accommodation too higher speeds without imposing too much strain on ill-adapted muscles and joints.

Toward the end of the program – when you have built up to around 5.5 MPH – you may find it easier to run than to walk. If you want to run, don't feel you have to hold back. If you can walk consistently at this speed, you are more than fit enough to run.

Resting: Progression (except in Fitness Categories 1 and 2) is from short bursts of effort to more sustained activity. The length of the resting period you should assume between bouts is up to you (the distance and calories expended will remain the same), but try to make it no more than one minute.

Frequency: Plan on doing at least 3 sessions a week: this is the minimum level at which the training effect (see p. 93) takes place. You can, of course, do more if you feel like it, and you will probably progress quicker; but your increase in fitness will probably not be commensurate with the increased time you put into your training.

Each individual session will make no great demands on you. You need no special clothing, there will be no pain, and the longest session is only 45 minutes. This may not sound like a lot, but even in Fitness Category 1, if you stick to the program, you will have covered 75 miles after 6 months.

Be flexible: Don't feel you have to stick rigidly to the category in which you first place yourself. You may find you adapt more quickly than you thought you would. If this is the case, simply promote yourself to the next category, slotting in at the equivalent level of calorie expenditure. For instance, weeks 12 to 14 of Fitness Category 1 are equivalent to weeks 7 and 8 of Category 2.

Age factor: Remember that for every decade over 30, the program should be stretched by 40 percent; this is because adaptation to the training load takes approximately 40 percent longer for each decade over 30. Again, there is no need to be rigid about this; simply repeat a week's schedule at regular intervals throughout the program to stretch it to the required amount.

Maintenance: After 6 months (or more if you're over 30), you should have reached a basic level of fitness. You should plan at least to maintain that level of fitness by walking, every week, the distance – and the pace – specified in the last week of your program. But there's no reason to stop there. You can work on through the categories and/or safely branch out into other sports.

Alternative approach: Instead of choosing a program and then finding a suitable walking area, you can, if you want to, use the opposite approach. Choose a walk you like; estimate its length; then time yourself over the distance comfortably. Match your speed and the distance to a suitable place in the program and build up from there.

If your walk has a few hills or slopes in it, so much the better. If you want to work out a more accurate calorie count, estimate an extra 3 calories per minute for ever 5 percent gradient.

DETERMINING YOUR FITNESS CATEGORY	
If your heart rate reaches training level over 440 yards (or paces) in:	Fitness Category
More than 5 mins. (less than 3 mph)	1
5 mins.–3 mins. 45 secs. (3.5–4.0 mph)	2
3 mins. 45 secs.–3 mins. 20 secs. (4.0–4.5 mph)	3
3 mins 20 secs.–3 mins. flat (4.5–5.0 mph)	4
Under 3 mins. (over 5.0 mph)	5

WALK!

Fitness Category 1

	Week	Approximate pace (mph)	Distance	Paces per minute	Repetitions per session	Total time (minutes)	Approx. calorie expenditure	Total distance per session (miles)
STARTER PROGRAM	1	3.00	1.50 miles	90	1	30	110	1.50
	2	3.50	1.50 miles	100	1	25	105	1.50
	3, 4	3.50	2.00 miles	100	1	34	143	2.00
	5, 6	3.50	2.50 miles	100	1	42	176	2.50
PROGRESSION	7, 8	3.75	2.50 miles	110	1	40	196	2.50
	9–11	3.75	2.75 miles	110	1	44	215	2.75
	12–14	4.00	2.75 miles	120	1	41	225	2.75
	15–18	4.00	3.00 miles	120	1	45	250	3.00
	19–22	4.25	3.00 miles	125	1	42	260	3.00
	23–26	4.25	3.25 miles	125	1	45	285	3.25
MAINTENANCE								

240

Fitness Category 2

	Week	Approxi-mate pace (mph)	Distance	Paces per minute	Repeti-tions per session	Total time (minutes)	Approx. calorie expenditure	Total distance per session (miles)
STARTER PROGRAM	1, 2	3.50	2.00 miles	100	1	35	143	2.00
	3, 1	4.00	2.00 miles	120	1	30	165	2.00
	5, 6	4.00	2.50 miles	120	1	38	206	2.50
PROGRESSION	7, 8	4.00	2.75 miles	120	1	41	225	2.75
	9, 10	4.25	2.75 miles	125	1	39	240	2.75
	11, 12	4.25	3.00 miles	125	1	42	260	3.00
	13, 14	4.50	3.00 miles	130	1	40	280	3.00
	15, 16	4.50	3.25 miles	130	1	43	300	3.25
	17, 18	4.00 / 4.50	110 yards / 220 yards	120 / 130	18	46	300	3.375
	19, 20	4.00 / 4.50	110 yards / 330 yards	120 / 130	13	42	300	3.25
	21, 22	4.00 / 4.50	110 yards / 440 yards	120 / 130	10	46	300	3.125
	23, 24	4.00 / 4.75	110 yards / 330 yards	120 / 135	13	45	310	3.25
	25, 26	4.00 / 4.75	110 yards / 440 yards	120 / 135	11	45	320	3.50
MAINTENANCE								

Fitness Category 3

	Week	Approxi- mate pace (mph)	Distance	Paces per minute	Repeti- tions per session	Total time (minutes)	Approx. calorie expenditure	Total distance per session (miles)
STARTER PROGRAM	1, 2	3.50 4.00	110 yards 110 yards	100 120	16	32	155	2.00
	3, 4	3.50 4.00	110 yards 220 yards	100 120	11	32	160	2.00
	5, 6	3.50 4.00	110 yards 330 yards	100 120	8	31	165	2.00
PROGRESSION	7, 8	3.75 4.00	110 yards 440 yards	110 120	7	37	175	2.18
	9, 10	3.75 4.00	110 yards 660 yards	110 120	6	38	200	2.62
	11, 12	3.75 4.50	110 yards 440 yards	110 132	8	34	220	2.50
	13, 14	3.75 4.50	110 yards 880 yards	110 132	4	30	205	2.25
	15, 16	3.75 4.75	110 yards 880 yards	110 138	4	28	210	2.25
	17, 18	4.00 4.75	440 yards 1 mile	120 138	2	33	240	2.50
	19, 20	4.00 5.00	440 yards 1 mile	120 145	2	31	240	2.50
	21, 22	4.00 5.00	660 yards 1 mile	120 145	2	35	260	2.75
	23, 24	4.00 5.00	1 mile 2 miles	120 145	1	40	280	3.00
	25, 26	5.00	3 miles	145	1	36	300	3.00
MAINTENANCE								

Fitness Category 4

	Week	Approxi-mate pace (mph)	Distance	Paces per minute	Repeti-tions per session	Total time (minutes)	Approx. calorie expenditure	Total distance per session (miles)
STARTER PROGRAM	1, 2	4.00 5.00	110 yards 220 yards	120 145	12	28	220	2.25
	3, 4	4.00 5.00	110 yards 330 yards	120 145	10	31	240	2.50
	5, 6	4.00 5.00	110 yards 440 yards	120 145	8	32	245	2.50
PROGRESSION	7, 8	4.00 5.00	110 yards 660 yards	120 145	6	33	260	2.60
	9, 10	4.50 5.00	110 yards 880 yards	132 145	5	34	280	2.80
	11, 12	4.50 5.00	440 yards ¾ mile	132 145	3	37	295	3.00
	13, 14	4.75 5.00	440 yards ¾ mile	138 145	3	37	295	3.00
	15, 16	4.75 5.25	660 yards ¾ mile	138 152	3	40	340	3.30
	17, 18	5.00 5.25	1 mile ¾ mile	145 152	2	44	375	3.50
	19, 20	5.00 5.50	¾ mile 1 mile	145 160	2	40	370	3.50
	21, 22	5.00 5.50	1.25 miles 2.5 miles	145 160	1	42	395	3.75
	23, 24	5.00 5.50	¾ mile 3 miles	145 160	1	42	405	3.75
	25, 26	5.50	4 miles	160	1	43	435	4.00
MAINTENANCE								

Fitness Category 5

	Week	Approxi-mate pace (mph)	Distance	Paces per minute	Repeti-tions per session	Total time (minutes)	Approx. calorie expenditure	Total distance per session (miles)
STARTER PROGRAM	1, 2	4.50 5.00	220 yards 220 yards	132 145	11	34	255	2.75
	3, 4	4.50 5.00	220 yards 440 yards	132 145	8	37	290	3.50
	5, 6	4.50 5.00	440 yards 880 yards	132 145	4	37	290	3.05
PROGRESSION	7, 8	4.50 5.50	550 yards 880 yards	132 160	4	38	340	3.25
	9, 10	4.75 5.50	550 yards 880 yards	138 145	4	37	345	3.25
	11, 12	5.00 5.50	1 mile ¾ mile	145 160	2	40	365	3.50
	13, 14	5.00 5.75	1 mile ¾ mile	160 170	2	40	370	3.50
	15, 16	5.25 5.75	¾ mile 1 mile	152 170	2	38	390	3.50
	17, 18	5.50 5.75	½ mile 1.5 miles	160 170	2	42	455	4.00
	19, 20	5.50 6.00	½ mile 1.5 miles	160 176	2	41	470	4.00
	21, 22	5.50 6.00	1.0 mile 3.0 miles	160 176	1	41	470	4.00
	23, 24	5.50 6.00	¾ mile 3.5 miles	160 176	1	43	500	4.25
	25, 26	6.00	4.5 miles	176	1	45	540	4.50
MAINTENANCE								

Appendix 4

Loosening Up: Some additional exercises to supplement the basic walking program

Walking builds foundation fitness; but as you work toward this level of fitness – and after you have achieved it – you may find you would like to build flexibility and strength in other ways. Here are some easy-to-do exercises that have been devised by fitness experts. They can be done at home, 3 to 5 times a week. They should take no more than 10–15 minutes in all. Don't force the pace to start with; later, when you feel fit enough, you can time yourself and use the exercises as an alternative means of raising your pulse.

> **Exercises 1–10 are quite easy.**
> **Exercises 11–14 are tougher and can be omitted initially.**

If you want to include a few more exercises, turn to pp. 71–2, which describe push-ups and sit-ups. These two exercises together are superb and dynamic additions to a full walking program. Simply tack them on to the end of the schedule outlined below.

---

1. TRUNK ROTATIONS

Purpose: To stretch muscles in the back, sides and shoulder girdle.

Movement: Stand astride; raise arms to shoulder level. Twist trunk to the right and arms to the left; avoid lifting your heels. Repeat 4 times, then repeat, twisting 4 times the other way.

Repetitions: 10 (i.e., 80 twists in all)

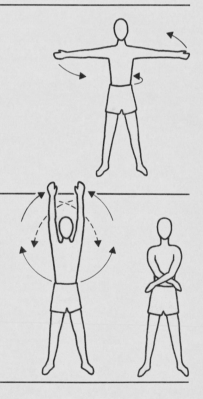

---

2. DOUBLE ARM CIRCLES AND TOE RAISES

Purpose: To stretch muscles of the shoulder girdle and to strengthen muscles of the feet.

Movement: Stand with feet about 12 inches apart and arms at sides. Swing arms up and around, making large circles. As arms are raised and crossed overhead, rise on toes.

Repetitions: 15

---

3. FORWARD BEND
Purpose: To stretch muscles of the buttocks and posterior leg.

Movement: Stand astride with hands on hips. Bend forward to a 90-degree angle; return to starting position; keep back flat.

Repetitions: 10

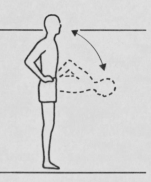

4. ABDOMINAL CHURN
Purpose: To stretch muscles of the buttocks, abdomen, and posterior leg.

Movement: Stand astride with hands on hips. Lower trunk sideways to left; rotate to forward position; return to upright position. Repeat and reverse direction after two rotations.

Repetitions: 10

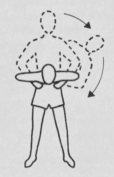

5. SHOULDER AND CHEST STRETCH
Purpose: To stretch muscles of the chest and shoulders.

Movement: Stand astride with arms at shoulder level and elbows bent. Force elbows backward and return to starting position.

Repetitions: 15

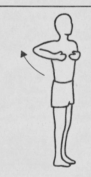

6. LOWER BACK STRETCH
Purpose: To stretch muscles in the lower back, buttocks and back of thigh.

Movement: Lie on back with the legs extended or stand erect. Lift and bend one leg; grasp the knee and keep the opposite leg flat; pull knee to chest. Repeat with alternate leg.

Repetitions: 20 (10 for each leg).

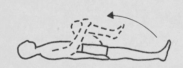

7. SIDE STRETCH

Purpose: To stretch the medial muscles of the thigh and the lateral muscles of the trunk and thorax.

Movement: Stand erect with one arm extended upward and the other relaxed at the side; place feet apart at more than shoulder width. Bend trunk directly to the right with the left arm stretching overhead; keep both feet flat. Use same procedure for other side.

Repetitions: 20 (10 for each side)

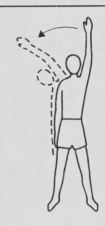

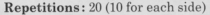

8. GROIN STRETCH

Purpose: To stretch the groin muscles.

Movement: Sit with knees bent outward and the bottoms of feet together. Grasp ankles and pull the upper body as close as possible to the feet.

Repetitions: 10

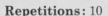

9. HAMSTRING STRETCH

Purpose: To stretch the muscles in the posterior leg and thigh.

Movement: Sit on ground with one leg extended straight forward; place the other leg forward with the knee bent and the sole touching the inner thigh of the extended leg. Bend forward and attempt to touch the head to the knee. Repeat with other leg.

Repetitions: 20 (10 for each leg)

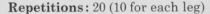

10. CALF STRETCHER

Purpose: To stretch the posterior leg muscles.

Movement: Stand in upright position with the balls of the feet on the edge of a step. Lower heels, then raise heels and rise on toes.

Repetitions: 10

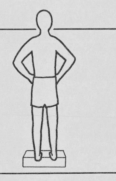

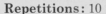

11. ADVANCED LOWER BACK AND HAMSTRING STRETCH

Purpose: To stretch muscles of the lower back and hamstring muscles.

Movement: Lie on back with legs bent. Keep knees together and slowly bring them over the head; straighten the legs and touch the toes to the floor; return to starting position. (As a variant, tuck the knees down by the ears. This loosens the neck marvelously but demands considerable flexibility, so don't force it.)

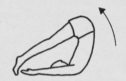

Repetitions: 10

12. INVERTED STRETCH

Purpose: To stretch and strengthen the anterior hip, buttocks, and abdominal muscles.

Movement: Sit with arms at side. Support body with heels and arms and raise trunk as high as possible.

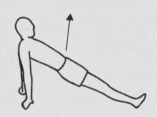

Repetitions: 10

13. FRONT LEG STRETCH

Purpose: To stretch the muscles of the anterior thigh and hip.

Movement: Lie on the ground with face down or stand erect. Pull the ankle to the hip slowly; hold for three seconds and release the ankle. Use same procedure for other side.

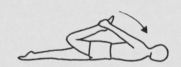

Repetitions: 20 (10 for each leg)

14. ADVANCED FRONT LEG STRETCH

Purpose: To stretch the muscles of the anterior thigh and leg.

Movement: Kneel with feet turned outward. Lean backward to touch ankles.

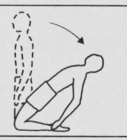

Repetitions: 10

Further Reading

Basic Fitness
Morehouse, Laurence E., and Leonard Gross. *Total Fitness in 30 Minutes A Week*. Hart-Davis, MacGibbon, London, 1975.
Pollock, Michael, Jack Wilmore and Samuel Fox. *Health and Fitness Through Physical Acitivity*. John Wiley & Sons, New York, 1978.

The Experience of Walking
Fletcher, Colin. *The Man Who Walked Through Time*. Vintage Books, New York, 1967.
Hillaby, John. *Journey Through Europe; Journey Through Britain; Journey Through Love; Journey to the Jade Sea* (all Paladin).
New York-New Jersey Trail Conference Inc. and The American Geographical Society. *New York Walk Book*. Doubleday/Natural History Press, New York, 1971.
Rudner, Ruth. *Off and Walking*. Holt, Rinehart and Winston, New York, 1977.
Sussman, Aaron and Ruth Goode. *The Magic of Walking*. Simon and Schuster, New York, 1967. Contains an extensive bibliography.

Backpacking
Fletcher, Colin. *The New Complete Walker*. Knopf, New York, 1974.
Hart, John. *Walking Softly in the Wilderness*. Sierra Club Books, San Francisco, 1977.
McManus, Patrick. *A Fine and Pleasant Misery*. Holt, Rinehart and Winston, New York, 1978.
New York-New Jersey Trail Conference. *The Official Guide to the Appalachian Trail*. The Appalachian Trail Conference, 1977.
Sharp, David. *Walking in the Countryside*. David & Charles, London 1978.

Nature Walking
The American Wilderness series, Time-Life Books, New York.
Hoskins, Professor W. G. *The Making of the English Landscape*. Penguin, 1977.
Terres, John. *The Walking Adventures of a Naturalist*. Hawthorn Books, Inc., New York, 1969.

Acknowledgments

This book draws on the expertise and advice of many people. In particular I would like to thank:

My publishers John and Janet Marqusee and editor Diane Flanel; Dr. Ian Anderson, London; Alan Blatchford and Chris Steed, Long Distance Walkers Association; Sophie Clarke-Jervoise; Susan de la Plain; Tim Fraser; Dr. Sam Fox, Georgetown Hospital, Washington; Gil Gleim, Institute of Sports Medicine and Athletic Trauma, New York; Arthur Gordon; Dr. Desmond and Sue Heath, New York; John Hillaby, Hampstead; Julian Hopkins, British race-walking coach; Sid Horenstein, American Museum of Natural History, New York; Sheila Kitzinger, Standlake, Oxfordshire; Paul Nihill, international race walker; Michael Pollock, Mt. Sinai Medical Center, Milwaukee, Wisconsin; Jean Porter, Audubon Sanctuary, Greenwich, Conn.; Dr. Richard Schuster, NY College of Podiatric Medicine; David Seymour, National Audubon Society; Dr. George Sheehan; Glen Swengros, President's Commission on Physical Fitness and Sport, Washington; Stewart Udall, Washington; Dr. John Waller, Hospital for Special Surgery, New York; George Zoebelein, Appalachian Trail Conference.

Picture Credits

The author and publishers wish to thank the following individuals and organizations for permission to reproduce their material:

Amateur Athletic Union of the United States: 221; Agricultural Hall, Islington, London (photo: John Goldblatt): 214; Lionel A. Atwill: 141; The Bettmann Archive: 15, 108–9, 119, 215; Ray Block: 10–11, 27, 31, 32–3 (all), 188–9, 192, 195, 199, 201, 203; John Goldblatt: 56–7, 214; John Hillaby: 231; Keystone Press: 87, 88, 220, 227, 228; Mark Mason: 6–7, 12–13, 28, 36–7, 84–5, 166–7, 174, 175, 177, 178–9 (all), 182; National Audubon Society Society: 66; Picturepoint, London: 140; Ramblers Association: 148, 150; *The Redditon Indicator and Alcester Chronicle*: 149; Royal Netherlands League for Physical Fitness, 217; Karen Sanders: 128, 129; Simon Schuster, Inc. (photo by Don Lordi): 39; Syndication International: 147; Wide World Photos: 52, 121, 122; UPI: 208–9.

Index

Page numbers in *italics* indicate illustrations.